LIGHTKEEPERS

The Power of Becoming Safe Harbour in the Mental Health Crisis

Mike Shoreman

Lightkeepers: The Power of Becoming Safe Harbour in the Mental Health Crisis
Copyright © Mike Shoreman, 2024.

No part of this publication may be reproduced, stored in a retrieval system, or transmitted in any form or by any means, electronic, mechanical, photocopying, recording, scanning, or otherwise, without the prior written permission of the author, except by reviewers, who may quote brief passages in a review.

To request permissions, contact the publisher at
jennifer@entouragemedia.ca.

ISBN (Paperback): 978–1–0689121–0–8
ISBN (Electronic book): 978–1–0689121–1–5

First Paperback Edition: October 2024

Printed in the USA
1 2 3 4 5 6 7 8 9 10

ENTOURAGE

Published by Entourage Media
www.entouragemedia.ca

Dedicated to all the ones who helped light the way.

CONTENTS

Foreword ix

Introduction xv

A Note About Language xix

Life by Design 1

Worst Case Scenario 15

Drowning 31

The Comeback | First Steps 41

Speaking | Innovation 57

Lake Ontario | Failure 87

Lake Erie | Team Support 103

Lake Huron | Lessons in Light 115

Lake Superior | Solution-Seeking 129

Lake Michigan | 4:1 Mental Health 153

Lake Ontario | Togetherness 167

Lighthouses 175

Epilogue 193

Resources 195

Acknowledgements 197

This story contains content about suicidal ideation. If you or someone you know is thinking about suicide, call or text 9-8-8. Help is available twenty-four hours a day, seven days a week. For more help, resources are available at the end of this book.

FOREWORD

Mike Shoreman's *Lightkeepers: The Power of Becoming Safe Harbour in the Mental Health Crisis* shines a light not only on stories of resilience and support, but also calls us all to be vigilant guides for those navigating rough psychological waters. Given our increasing social awareness of the role of mental well-being, the role of a "Lightkeeper" has never been more crucial.

Across Canada, we have never needed attention to mental health as much as we do now. Every year, one in five Canadians experiences mental health challenges. By the time Canadians reach forty years of age, one in two will have a current or past mental illness.[1] Recent research shows that rates of mental health conditions have significantly increased in the last decade, with one in three not having access to services to address those

---

1   Smetanin et al. (2011). The life and economic impact of major mental illnesses in Canada: 2011-2041. Prepared for the Mental Health Commission of Canada. Toronto: RiskAnalytica.

needs.[2] One of the most tragic outcomes of pain and distress is suicide. In Canada, there are approximately 4,500 deaths by suicide per year, or approximately twelve people per day.[3] We know that suicide is preventable, but that means we must shore up our efforts at prevention.

This is particularly true for youth, who are at the beginning of their life journey. However, more youth than ever are struggling. The recent Ontario Student Drug Use and Health Survey (OSDUHS) brought to light the declining mental health of youth. More than half of students surveyed indicated a moderate-to-serious level of psychological distress, a figure that has doubled over the past decade. One in five students report harming themselves on purpose, and one in six had serious thoughts about suicide in the past year.[4] There is an opportunity to intervene to create a better supported and more resilient pathway for youth development.

Mike's deep commitment stems from personal experience and strength that has grown with each challenge. He understands the ebbs and flows of mental health struggles—the moments when the waters are calm and those when they are

---

2 Statistics Canada. Mental Disorders in Canada, 2022. https://www150.statcan.gc.ca/n1/pub/11-627-m/11-627-m2023053-eng.htm

3 Statistics Canada. Suicide in Canada: Key Statistics. https://www.canada.ca/en/public-health/services/publications/healthy-living/suicide-canada-key-statistics-infographic.html

4 CAMH. The Ontario Student Drug Use and Health Survey (OSDUH). https://www.camh.ca/en/science-and-research/institutes-and-centres/institute-for-mental-health-policy-research/ontario-student-drug-use-and-health-survey---osduhs

tumultuous and foreboding. This understanding continues to lead him to act on behalf of others who are struggling.

Imagine a lighthouse standing tall against the stormy skies that often cloak the Great Lakes, an apt metaphor for Mike's endurance and his mission. Lighthouses serve a singular purpose: to illuminate and guide. Much like these steadfast structures, Mike's journey on a paddleboard across the vast and unpredictable expanses of the Great Lakes is both symbolic and transformative. Every wave surmounted symbolizes the challenges faced by individuals struggling with mental health issues, yet most importantly, each stroke of the paddle against the water echoes perseverance and hope.

In *Lightkeepers*, Mike invites us into the world where he dedicates himself to being a beacon, particularly for youth who often find themselves adrift without a clear course. Here, the role of Lightkeeper extends beyond just providing guidance; it is about creating a safe harbour, a place where one can find respite, solidarity, and strength to set sail once again.

As a Lightkeeper himself, Mike Shoreman is attuned to the subtle and overt signals of distress, guiding others with compassion and actionable wisdom. Lighthouses also symbolize connection—a bridge between the relentless sea and the safety of land. Similarly, Mike's work builds bridges between individuals and communities, fostering an environment where those battling mental health issues are seen, heard, and supported. By igniting discussions and bringing mental health into the realm of everyday conversation, he helps dismantle stigma, allowing light to pierce through the obscurity of misunderstanding and isolation.

What is perhaps most remarkable about *Lightkeepers* is its call to the reader. Mike's message is a clarion call for us all to become Lightkeepers in our own circles. Whether family members, friends, or colleagues, we are moved to adopt the mindset of a lighthouse: steadfast, illuminating, and inclusive. The book serves as a reminder that in the rough, unpredictable waters of mental health, even a single light can change the course of one's journey.

As the Chief Medical Officer for 9-8-8: Suicide Crisis Helpline, this action to raise awareness, defeat stigma, and build community through connection resonates deeply with our own mission. 9-8-8: Suicide Crisis Helpline launched across Canada in November 2023. Available to people of all ages, by phone and text, twenty-four hours per day, in English and French, this service is a resource for those thinking about suicide or for anyone who is concerned about someone. Responders on 9-8-8 create non-judgemental support and connection. In the first year of service, 9-8-8 has already received approximately one thousand calls and texts per day. Mike has been an ardent advocate and supporter of 9-8-8.

In embracing the role of a Lightkeeper, one not only helps others but also embarks on a personal journey of growth and self-awareness. Through supporting others, we discover our capacities for empathy and kindness, much as a lighthouse continually withstands the elements, providing an unwavering signal of hope and direction.

As you delve into *Lightkeepers*, may you be inspired by Mike Shoreman's courageous heart and transformative insight. May you find within its pages not only solace and empowerment but also the motivation to become a beacon in your own right. Together, we can guide each other towards safer harbours and welcoming shores, and thus ensure that no one is left to navigate life's waters alone.

Allison Crawford, MD, PhD
Psychiatrist and Chief Medical Officer of 9-8-8: Suicide Crisis Helpline
Professor, Departments of Psychiatry and Dalla Lana School of Public Health
University of Toronto

INTRODUCTION

You can find light in the most extraordinary of places. I learned this in the middle of the Great Lakes on a cold, black night, with my hands shaking so violently I could barely hold onto my paddle.

My body had used up every ounce of energy, and I still had another fifteen minutes before my next liquid meal. If I was going to make this fourth (of five) crossing and not let everyone down, I didn't have time to stop. Every time I took a break for a minute or two, the wind and waves pushed me backward, sentencing me to make up the distance lost.

Exhaustion had taken on a new meaning after twenty-one hours of paddling. It would have been so easy to simply slide off my board and rest my screaming muscles. Of course, that would've also meant sinking beneath the surface of Lake Michigan, and I wasn't about to give up.

I was there, against all odds, to put out a call to action as loudly as I could. I wanted to ring the alarm and create change for millions of others who couldn't do so for themselves *because they were me, only a couple of years beforehand.*

We are in a mental health crisis. As Allison Crawford wrote in her foreword, one in five Canadians will experience a mental health challenge this year. In the US, the numbers aren't any better.

Studies and numbers help put the crisis in perspective, but let's also put them in context. These numbers represent people, the true stories of millions of people in North America. They tell me that one in five of my friends, family, colleagues, and neighbours could be suffering from an invisible, sometimes debilitating illness.

At the same time, only one in three people who reported having mental health illness reported seeking treatment for it.[5]

Thanks to the centuries-old stigma of shame surrounding mental health, admitting to struggling can feel like opening oneself up to misunderstanding, judgment, or rejection.

When someone close to us asks, "How are you?" our first response is often, "Good, thanks," no matter how we feel. Shining a light on personal mental health struggles can be uncomfortable.

So, what would happen if we looked at the one-in-five statistic in a different way? What if we turned the spotlight around,

---

5 "The State of Mental Health in Canada - CCLA." 2017. CCLA. February 9, 2017. https://ccla.org/get-informed/talk-rights/the-state-of-mental-health-in-canada/?gad_source=1&gclid=Cj0KCQjwrKu2BhDkARIsAD7GBovEIcqhB0p5QRIuwp-WVH946X-hOPz2-ACDeb1-WElsIxxCf2wer48saAuAJEALw_wcB.

INTRODUCTION

taking it off the one person who is struggling and lighting up the other four, empowering them to show up in a different way?

Canada has the world's longest coastline and more lakes than the rest of the world combined. It is home to more than 750 lighthouses and long-range lights, fifty-one of which are staffed by "Lightkeepers."

Lightkeepers serve many purposes, ranging from issuing tsunami warnings off the North Pacific coast to offering search-and-rescue services and sanctuary to those in need. Lighthouses "keep the light," shining a beacon to mark dangerous coastlines, reefs, and shallow areas and guide ships to safe harbour.[6]

Imagine if we could all be Lightkeepers, offering sanctuary in the storm for friends, loved ones, neighbours, and colleagues who might otherwise feel isolated, scared, or unable to ask for help.

Then, take that idea a step further.

Imagine putting this same system into effect within the current non-profit and government mental health organizations that already exist.

My story is a familiar one: I'm not the first to have the rug pulled out from beneath them, suffer a mental health breakdown, or be told my debilitating disabilities are forever. So how is this story ever going to stand out enough to create change and leave an imprint?

---

6   Canada,. 2024. "Lighthouses in Canada." Dfo-Mpo.gc.ca. 2024. https://www.dfo-mpo.gc.ca/otw-am/lighthouses-phares/canada-eng.html#2.

Simple.

You and I are going to give it a new ending.

Together.

Yours truly,
Mike Shoreman

A NOTE ABOUT LANGUAGE

Words matter. Language evolves to adapt to new information and to rid us of old biases. Mental health and mental illness are often used interchangeably, but they are not the same thing. Like physical health, mental health refers to a state of well-being. Mental health includes our emotions, feelings of connection to others, our thoughts and feelings, and being able to manage life's highs and lows. The presence or absence of a mental illness is not a predictor of mental health; someone without a mental illness could have poor mental health, just as a person with a mental illness could have excellent mental health. Everyone will experience challenges regarding their mental well-being, but not everyone will experience a mental illness.

CHAPTER 1

LIFE BY DESIGN

As the plane lifted off the tarmac and began its climb toward the sun, I couldn't wipe the smile off my face. And that's saying something for someone who just made their way through the madness of the LAX.

I looked out my little window, which was soon filled with a view of the incredible California coastline below. I tried to pick out the beach where I would be spending half the year, but there were too many inlets and shores below to identify which one was about to be mine. I imagined surfers, swimmers, and paddleboarders in the ocean below and already wished I were back down there with them.

The pilot was saying something on the crackly PA system about our destination and the weather or something else, but all I could focus on was how much my life was about to change.

It was the last week of October 2018, and I was an early-thirty-something entrepreneur with big ideas for my business.

I wanted to be in control of my future, to live a life by my own design—and, of course, make enough money to live comfortably.

It never occurred to me to work a desk job. Not for the long run, at least. I liked—needed—to be active. I enjoyed playing just about any sport I could, any chance I got, whether I was any good at it or not.

When I wasn't doing that, I was watching sports from the stands or on television. Luckily, since my hometown of Toronto was home to the Leafs, Jays, Raptors, and Argonauts, there was no shortage of ways to immerse myself in sports whenever I wanted to.

I remember when I first got into paddleboarding. Not only was it a good workout (even on a calm day), but it was also unlike any other activity. Sometimes, it would just be me and a friend paddling with the sunset on one side of us and the skyline behind us. Other times, it was an afternoon of exploration. There was always something to discover. I remember paddling to a bird sanctuary where the flock allowed us to float through and around them. No matter what, paddleboarding was always an adventure and always beautiful.

Pretty much right after my first time on a board, I bought my own and began spending countless summer days on Lake Ontario, paddling between the beaches and the island. One board became two, then more. Soon, I was certified and helped other beachgoers get into paddleboarding. I gave lessons and rented out my extra boards for group excursions. By my second summer, it was a full-time, seasonal business, and I'd never been happier. The money was good, too—good enough to support a life in Toronto, which is known to be one of Canada's most expensive cities.

I spent pretty much every day on the water, to the point that my friends began to complain they never saw me anymore. They were used to the version of me who was the first of their friends to show up. Want to dance all night at a new club? I was in! New restaurant? Yes. Catch a musical? Absolutely.

I loved that version of me, too, but because I could clearly see the future I was shaping for myself, it took priority over everything else.

"If you want to see me, come to the beach!" I said.

And thankfully, they did!

Whenever my friends wanted to hang out, they'd grab their boards (or use mine), meet me on the shore, and we'd spend hours on the water, chatting and exploring the lake—sometimes with my clients, sometimes in between lessons. With paddleboarding, more people equals more fun.

Those hangout sessions on the lake are still some of my favourite memories.

Basically, I ate, slept, and breathed the paddleboard business. I woke up excited to get out on the water each day. It was all I could do to force breakfast down my throat before grabbing my boards and heading out.

Sometimes, I would take one or two people (or clients) out on the boards and do some lessons; other times groups of six or more for a group excursion. We'd paddle out into the lake, ending up between the Toronto islands and the city, with planes going back and forth overhead . . . There was nothing else like it.

I was lucky that my clientele ranged from beginners and bachelorette parties to television media personalities. One day, I found myself taking out US figure skating Olympian Jason Brown. He was training in Toronto with Brian Orser at the time. I remember thinking, "What is my life?"

I was building a career I loved and achieving some of my biggest dreams.

The problem was that once October came around, the lake grew cold and put an end to paddleboarding, cutting my months of operation in half.

And it was October again.

I heard a chime echo through the cabin of the plane, indicating that we could take our seat belts off and relax for the rest of the five-hour flight from LA to Toronto.

My head had begun to pound, first while going through the airport, and now as we flew above the clouds.

Must be from excitement. Or stress. Or both.

I ordered a sugar-free cola from a flight attendant pushing a cart of snacks and beverages and fished two extra-strength painkillers out of my bag.

My mind was flooded with all the things I wanted to plan and do in the weeks ahead. Everything was about to change.

Even though the week on the West Coast had been exhilarating, visiting Laguna Beach wasn't a vacation. It was research. I was there to explore a partnership with another company that also did water sports lessons and rentals. The potential partner and I had spent the week talking business, taking boards out on the ocean, and making plans for the winter ahead. The more we talked and planned, the more everything clicked into place. It was going to work.

The plan was to operate my business as usual until November. Then, while lake-water temperatures plummeted as winter approached (in November, the average temperature would be eight to ten degrees Celsius), I'd operate in California. This partnership meant turning my six-month business into a year-round one.

The bright sunshine coming in through the window seemed to make my head hurt a bit more, but closing the shade felt criminal on such a gorgeous day. Instead, I closed my eyes. It took nearly an hour to calm my adrenaline and excitement down enough to fall asleep, but once I was out, I was *out*. It wasn't until the sweet southern flight attendant squeezed my shoulder a few times that I came back to reality.

The headache was still there, but I didn't care. All I could think about was getting through Pearson Airport, getting home, parking myself at my desk, and getting started on planning and logistics for the new partnership. It would literally double my business. I didn't want to waste any time.

* * *

It was the first week of November, and my cup of tea felt warm in my hands as I cradled it and surveyed the list of tasks on the screen. There was a lot I wanted to get organized before I could return to California to soak up as much of the season as possible. November had officially just arrived, and with it, cold temperatures on the lake. In another eight to twelve weeks, Lake Ontario would be mostly covered in ice.

My eyes felt strangely hot, and my head hurt. *How long have I been staring at the screen?* I tried turning down the brightness, but it didn't offer any relief.

This headache was not letting up. It had been bothering me off and on since my flight. *This must be what migraines feel like.* Luckily, I'd never had one before. In fact, I'd never really been sick with anything—no allergies or illnesses other than a broken arm at ten years old after a fluke accident.

I took a couple of painkillers and got up from the desk to stretch out my stiff muscles. After twelve-hour days of physical activity all summer, my body was *not* happy with hours and hours of computer work.

I stood there for a moment, debating how to fit in some activity before going back to the computer now that it was getting close to noon. My mind felt fuzzy, as if my tea had been spiked.

All of a sudden, the room's walls and ceiling started to spin. *What the hell?* It moved slowly at first and then faster, escalating in speed until my stomach started to turn with it. The floor also started to move to one side, slanting as if I were in a fun house at a carnival (this was definitely *not* fun), threatening to take me with it. I grasped for the arm of the couch nearby for support. My legs felt weak, as if I had just run a marathon, but I managed to stay upright. I don't know how long it took, but the walls and floor of my basement office eventually returned to their rightful place, and I let out a breath I didn't know I'd been holding.

Okay, that was . . . weird.

That's when a wave of exhaustion hit me like a truck. My plans for getting some exercise felt like a distant dream. A nap sounded much more realistic. I sank gratefully down onto the couch and stretched out. Despite my pounding head and concern over the random dizzy spell, I fell asleep within seconds.

***

Somewhere in the room, my cell phone chirped with message notifications. I had a vague feeling it had been doing that for quite some time. There was a glow from my laptop on the desk but otherwise, it was dark in the office and outside the window.

Have I slept all day?!

I never crashed that hard. Especially not when there was so much I wanted to get done.

I thought about California and bolted upright, ready to jump back into work. But that's about as far as I got. A sharp, stabbing pain pierced my ear from out of nowhere. I instinctually covered my ear with my hand and realized it felt a bit puffy to the touch. *Did I pick up a cold or flu on the trip?* I thought of the headache I'd been fending off since the plane ride, which started making sense now.

Okay, let's triage, I thought. I hadn't eaten in forever. I barely touched my tea. And I definitely needed more pain medication. But before I could even move again, the thought of doing much of anything felt inexplicably impossible. My body felt heavy and strange. The more I tried to think, the more my ear hurt.

I slowly laid back down, avoiding any contact between my ear and the surface of the couch and pillows. Sleep took over again.

The next day, it was pain that woke me up, not phone notifications. Any hopes for healing in my sleep evaporated. My ear was screaming. And throbbing. *That can't be good.* Without thinking, I got up and was instantly pushed back down, this time by an overwhelming feeling of nausea. The room was spinning again, but slower this time.

I used the furniture landmarks—coffee table, printer table, support column—to grab onto or lean on to help me get to the bathroom in one piece. Once my feet hit the cool tile of the bathroom floor, I delivered yesterday's meals into the toilet.

Throwing up made my ear hurt more. It had become a searing hot pain. I gripped the sink and the toilet to keep me grounded. The floor had begun to move again. This was going to require more than some over-the-counter medication and rest.

I needed a doctor.

It was November 5.

* * *

At a nearby walk-in clinic, I described my symptoms to a doctor who glanced in my ear, had me open up and say "ah," and asked me how long I had been feeling like this, if I'd been travelling, et cetera.

I told the doctor about paddleboarding in California.

"You most likely have an ear infection from getting dirty water in your ear," the doctor said, writing notes on my chart. He gave me a prescription for antibiotics and a more powerful pain medication.

I went home, took my medication as directed, and waited for the pain, dizziness, and vomiting to go away. It didn't.

As the day went on, my nausea and pain increased in severity.

I wanted to believe it was just an ear infection. I hoped

for relief, but the more I threw up, the weaker I became. I wasn't able to eat or drink anything. What little I did take in just came back up as soon as the room started to spin again—which seemed to happen anytime I opened my eyes. So, I slept a lot.

My ear was now twice the normal size. It throbbed in sync with my heartbeat.

My body's alarms were all going off at once, and I knew I had to listen. I dragged myself to my car, got in, and pointed it toward the nearest hospital. It wasn't a long drive, but within a few minutes, the lines on the road started to blur. *That's not good.* Dread set in with the reality of how serious this was. I tried to focus on simply not driving off the road.

The process of going from waiting room to triage nurse to ER to seeing a doctor took about three and a half hours, which is average for a hospital in Ontario.

My doctor was young and spoke fast: "I see you are having some ear pain. How long has that been happening? Let me take a look."

He didn't ask me about the nausea, vertigo, or weakness.

He looked in my ear and scanned the medical chart from the walk-in clinic I'd been to a couple of days before.

He saw I was already diagnosed with an ear infection from swimming in California and closed my chart. "Yes, it looks like you have an ear infection."

I didn't realize until later that this was clearly medical

anchoring bias: the tendency to perceptually lock on to salient features in the patient's initial presentation too early in the diagnostic process and then, worse, fail to adjust this initial impression in the light of later information. Nearly synonymous with confirmation bias.

"Are you sure? The meds aren't working, and this feels so much worse than an ear infection. In fact, everything seems to be getting much worse."

I squinted against the fluorescent lights of the busy ward. The light was harsh, making my eyes burn and my head pound louder.

"Yes, you just need to give the medication time to work," he said. "I'll give you another prescription for different antibiotics and some medication to help manage the pain. That should help."

No scans. No tests.

This time, I went to my mom's instead, where she could keep an eye on me.

I didn't know what else to do but listen to the doctor. Because the pain was so bad, I began taking more medication more often. I would have done just about anything to get even a fraction of relief. I continued to suffer despite the new prescriptions but felt better knowing my mom was nearby if things went off the rails.

"Jesus, Mike," my dad said when he came to check on me. He was shocked to see the state I was in. I could tell that he was distraught by my appearance. I don't remember much of what he said.

* * *

The next day, I woke up in a fog. The walls of the bedroom looked wrong somehow. I stared at them for a moment before the world fell back into context, and I remembered I was at my mother's house. Everything felt strange, including my body. I shuffled down the stairs, trying not to fall, fighting the dizziness. I was getting used to being dizzy but not getting any better and manoeuvring through it.

I'll never forget the look on my mother's face when she saw me.

"Mike!" she gasped.

"Wha—"

"Your face!" she whispered and got up from her chair.

"Why are you looking at me like that?!" I asked although I'm not sure any sound actually came out of my mouth. If she explained, I didn't hear her. I pointed myself toward the bathroom and got there just in time to heave into the toilet.

"Mike, we're going to the hospital. That last one obviously had no idea what they were doing."

She was moving around the house as I gripped the toilet. I heard her keys jingle.

"I think you might have had a stroke. Oh my God," she

said, mostly to herself. I could tell she was panicking. And now I was, too.

What was she talking about? I clumsily flushed and went to the sink to wash my hands. That's when I saw it. Saw me.

My face.

CHAPTER 2

WORST CASE SCENARIO

I stared at my face in the mirror—but it was more like a partially collapsed, abstract version of my face. My left eye was drooping, and one side of my mouth had fallen. I tried to blink and couldn't. I tried to fix my mouth and couldn't.

It was as if the painter of my features accidentally spilled water down one half of the canvas and just left me that way.

"Holy shit," I exclaimed, but it came out more like "Ho shhhttt."

I had only seen faces like that on people who'd had strokes before. "No!" This couldn't be happening. "No, no, no, no, no." I was too young.

My mom came up behind me and said, "We have to go *now*."

I covered my face with my hands as we drove. I didn't want people in the cars beside us or those waiting at crosswalks to see me looking like this.

Mom pulled her car into the circular driveway of the Emergency entrance of a different hospital, one hour away. I pulled the hood of my sweater forward over my face and got out of the car, wishing no one was there to see me.

"Just wait here and I'll come in with you," she promised and disappeared to find parking. She was probably calling my father, too, so that he knew what was going on.

I awkwardly leaned against a column of the entrance and stared at the ground.

My stomach was doing somersaults, warning me it was time to throw up again. *Please, no.* But I already knew it was too late. I barely made it to the grass before I threw up all over it in front of the people walking by and in full view of the nurses in the triage centre.

Having seen my grotesque display, a nurse came out to rescue me. She gave me a bunch of tissues to wipe my mouth with and, thankfully, a bag to throw up again. The nurse ushered me inside to get checked out. There was no long waiting period this time. Someone took me through the waiting room and into the ER bays within ten minutes.

"You're definitely dehydrated," said the nurse.

Made sense. It was November 11, and I'd been vomiting for six days straight by that point. But I knew there had to be more to it.

"Let's give you some IV fluids and see how you do." Her confidence temporarily took the edge off my fear.

For several hours, I was hooked up to an IV. I covered my face as best as I could whenever someone walked by. I impatiently waited for an explanation, or tests, or something—anything—that would explain what was going on.

With hydration, I'll admit, I felt a lot better, but something was still seriously wrong. All you had to do was look at me to see that.

The doctor came in with my chart in hand, gave me a ten-second look-over, and said, "Let's send you home with an IV of fluids and antibiotics. A nurse will come to your house each day to check on you and switch out your medication. That should help get your ear infection under control."

Go home? Seriously?

I couldn't believe the words coming out of his mouth.

"What about Mike's facial features?" I heard my mom demand. "Why does it look as if he's had a stroke?"

Once again, there were no scans or tests run. How could they know what was wrong with me?

"Infections can do all sorts of things. You'd be surprised," the doctor said, making it sound as if ear infections cause facial paralysis all the time. "Let's give the medication time to combat this ear infection. These antibiotics are much stronger. If your symptoms don't improve by the second day of home care, I want you to come back to the hospital."

So, once again, I did what I was told and went home. A home nurse came to see me and switch out my IV medication.

My face remained the same while the rest of my symptoms grew worse. I could barely walk or talk.

By the second day, my body was shaking from exhaustion and my pain had gone from excruciating to off the charts.

My mom took me to a *third* hospital since the symptoms had begun over a week prior.

"We have to get to the bottom of this. You can barely walk," she said.

This time, the hospital didn't take the ear infection diagnosis as the final word. They ran blood work and gave me my *first* CT scan, which, given the circumstances—my face had partially collapsed!—was unbelievable.

When the results came back, it was a specialist who delivered the answer. He took a seat on a black pleather-topped swivel stool and faced my mom and me.

With a deep breath, he explained, "We are dealing with a very rare condition called Ramsay Hunt syndrome." He put his clipboard down on a nearby table and looked at me. His face was friendly but grim. I didn't take that as a good sign.

"What's that?" asked Mom.

"Ramsay Hunt syndrome is a rare neurological disorder that is caused when the previously inactive or dormant varicella-zoster virus is reactivated. That's the same virus that causes chickenpox in children and shingles in adults. It only affects five in one hundred thousand people. What makes it even more rare is that this ordinarily affects adults over sixty years of age. And you're half that age."

I could barely register the words of the specialist through the shroud of exhaustion and excruciating pain.

"But *why* does it look like he's had a stroke?!" my mom pushed, motioning to my face in exasperation. "And why is he so nauseous? How can he be this sick from chicken pox?"

"The disorder is characterized by facial weakness or paralysis of the facial nerve. You've probably heard it referred to as facial palsy. It also comes with a rash affecting the ear or mouth, which is probably why the first doctor you saw assumed you had an ear infection."[7]

He went on to explain that it was attacking my ear, vestibular system, and my equilibrium. Symptoms are usually on one side of the face (unilateral). Ringing in the ears (tinnitus) and hearing loss were usually also present. "All of that together can create extreme vertigo. That's why Mike is having such trouble with mobility and balance."

It was hard to comprehend the information coming at me. I hoped my mom was getting more of it than I was.

"Let's get you off the antibiotics. You seem to be having a reaction to them. And let's try to reduce the pain and swelling of your nerves with some anti-inflammatories."

"And my face?" I gestured in frustration to my collapsed facial features.

---

7   "Ramsay Hunt Syndrome." 2024. National Organization for Rare Disorders. July 25, 2024. https://rarediseases.org/rare-diseases/ramsay-hunt-syndrome/.

Even as the room spun, I could tell that the specialist was choosing his words carefully.

"Some patients may have permanent facial paralysis or hearing loss, but that doesn't mean that will happen in your case."

Did he just say permanent?

"There *is* usually a good prognosis when treatment is started within three days of the onset of symptoms. However, we are on day ten."

"The doctors just kept telling him it was an ear infection," my mom said angrily. I could tell that she was trying to remain calm for me. She avoided my gaze.

The doctor continued, "Mike is young. And now that we know what it is, we can treat it much more effectively."

The doctor was talking in *maybes* and *ifs* in terms of my ability to smile, talk, and walk. That was not okay. This couldn't be it. Two weeks ago, I was fine. More than fine. I was playing in the surf at the location of my new winter business. How could things have changed so drastically so fast?

The only thing that brought me a small feeling of safety was that this doctor was taking me seriously.

* * *

Within a few more days, my speech became more affected. I couldn't close my left eye because the lid was paralyzed, and so it became irritated. Eventually, I started to lose vision in my eye.

The vertigo continued to spiral out of control. If I was awake, I was almost always violently ill. I had to carry a bucket or big bowl around with me wherever I went since there was no guarantee I'd make it to the bathroom in time.

Daily life changed dramatically. I went from spending days on the water to planning my schedule around an array of appointments.

To rule out brain damage, I had a number of MRIs. Because of my symptoms, each appointment took a lot of energy and preparation. Afterward, I would go home immediately and crash.

The weakness and exhaustion I experienced were shocking. I didn't know someone could feel that tired. Days blurred into one another.

I was too sick to make meals for myself and too tired to care if I ate or not.

Quickly, it was established that I needed *a lot* of care, and it wouldn't be easy.

My mom and dad, who'd been divorced since I was two years old, selflessly decided to share the workload of my care between the two of them.

They'd been apart for so long that I didn't have a single memory of them together.

Throughout my childhood, I'd always had two Christmases, two houses, and two separate families. At my dad's, we ate home-cooked meals, which was nice. But it was always a bit awkward for me. I felt as if I had to try to fit in with his second wife and her kids. I often felt like a fish out of water. It's like every other weekend, I would walk into this other family and try to find my place within it. Then I'd leave and go back to my other home.

My mom's parenting style was more relaxed. I grew up faster there. She treated me more like an adult, a friend. We would go out to eat together, order fast food, watch *Beverly Hills 90210* and then *Melrose Place* together (before binge-watching was possible, of course). Life with Mom was easier and more comfortable. She is hilarious. We both are, especially when we're together. We share the same sense of humour.

My dad is funny too, but usually when you don't expect it. He'll say something in the middle of a conversation and you're like, "Wait. What did you say?!" And we'd all burst out laughing. He's a character. He once learned the guitar just because he had family coming over and thought it would be fun to play for them. I remember asking him if he was nervous. He just laughed and said "no" because he said there would be drinking, so most wouldn't remember how he did anyway.

My dad was there for me in different ways, and I was okay with that. He was the one who took me to Quebec and stayed in the hotel, essentially on his own, while I went off to the lake each day to be certified in paddleboarding instruction. Here was someone who dropped everything to drive me to a different province just to be sure that I had what I needed to start a new career. To say that I'm lucky to have the parents that I do is an understatement.

* * *

As Mom and Dad split the workload of nursing me back to health (or trying to), it meant spending ten days at my mom's, then ten days at my dad's, on rotation. This way, each of them got to have a physical and emotional rest to recharge and still have a social life. Plus, we thought the change of scenery would be good for me.

I know that helping me get through the days and to all my appointments was an all-consuming job. I don't know what I would've done without their help.

Being so entirely dependent on my parents re-confirmed how different my life and prospects looked.

Despite the full-time help and numerous doctors and specialists, it felt like no matter what any of us did, I saw very little improvement. I was still violently off-balance nearly all the time. Even the smallest routine activities were difficult, if not impossible.

By early December, I began to come to terms with the fact that this was the best it was going to get. I stopped interacting with people. Messages filled my phone with encouragement and love: "You've got this, Mike"; "It'll get better!"; "Keep me in the loop," and offers of help. But I didn't want them to see me. And I knew there was nothing they could do to help. Not really.

From somewhere beneath my blanket of depression, I knew each message translated to "I love you," but the thought of faking positivity to alleviate other people's worry only added to my existing exhaustion.

I knew people wanted updates on my progress. I didn't know how to tell them there weren't any.

All the prospects of a future I'd designed myself had been blown up by this random illness. I found myself crying for the loss of my future. I knew there was more to life than appearances, but I missed the polished version of the guy I was used to seeing in my reflection. Gone were the days of the three-week haircut, using hair products, or taking the time it took to look the part of who I thought I was.

It was as if I were in the woods with a fire that would soon simmer and die, leaving me in the dark with no way to find my way and no way to light the torch again.

I tried to envision a future without hope of improvement, one in which *this* was how I would always be—dizzy, violently ill, with a broken-looking face, loss of speech, sight, and hearing, barely able to walk, barely able to look in the mirror, no money, no career . . . It broke me.

***

Christmas was approaching, and I went into it with the idea that it would be the last one I'd have with my family. I planned to be gone soon.

When my mom was at work, I sold my truck (which I loved) for $300 to a scrap metal dealer so I could afford Christmas gifts. Watching a stranger drive it away was one of the most defeating moments of my life, but there was no point in keeping it. I wasn't going to need a truck much longer.

I also sold my paddleboards. I couldn't walk, much less balance on a paddleboard. I didn't want my family to have to deal with them, so I posted them for sale online. I was out of the house at one appointment or another when the buyer came and picked them up off the porch. No ceremony. No handshake. Just my most loved possessions, gone. It was soul-crushing and somehow also a relief. One less thing to worry about.

Selling my possessions was just one of several milestones reminding me *I was on my way out*. Done with normal life, my business, my autonomy . . .

On social media and at home, my friends and family were celebrating the holidays. I had always been a huge Christmas person. I loved decorating the tree, giving presents, playing board games (Monopoly and Trivial Pursuit were big in our family), cards, wearing ugly Christmas sweaters and those silly paper crowns from used Christmas crackers.

By then, I was a shell of who I used to be. I went through the motions with the people I loved in rooms filled with holiday traditions, hugs, gifts, laughter, and love. I avoided looking anyone in the eyes. I didn't want them to see the nerve damage in my face any more than necessary. I hated that I needed a cane just to walk from one room to the next.

Once the holidays were over, I mentally checked out of my life, knowing the end was near. My dad and I were at an appointment, and the specialist suggested that vestibular therapy could help alleviate my vertigo and bring my balance back. I had given up hope for answers, but Dad was excited for any prospect of improvement.

"We could try to get you started in March," the doctor told me.

"No, if this can help, you'll get him started *today*," Dad declared. He wasn't going to take no for an answer. And he didn't. He took me to a private clinic and told them, "I want you to treat my son right away," and they did.

My dad is the kind of person you want to have on your side in a crisis.

I have no idea what it cost, but I think my dad sensed how close to the end I was and saw this as a way to bring me back.

Vestibular therapy was a weekly appointment he personally took me to. It was one of the only times I left my house by then. The exercises seemed so simple, yet for me, they were next to impossible, which made me angry with myself. I was coached to walk, very slowly, down a corridor with one of my hands on the wall. As I took my steps, I was to move my head up and down, or side to side, also while holding my cane with the other hand. Every time I moved my head, I felt dizzy. The idea was that the exercise would help me reprogram my brain and regain equilibrium so I could walk in a straight line again.

It was frustrating. I must have looked like a drunk person staggering their way through a sobriety test.

Over the first month, then the second, I saw little to no progress from the new therapy. In fact, there was no promise I would see any progress at all. I heard the phrase, "Let's see how it goes," a *lot*.

Despite failure and frustration at my own inabilities, I found myself liking my vestibular therapist, Shane. He had a nice smile, kind eyes, and was compassionate. He was a sports fan like me, so we chatted and connected over a shared interest in hockey, baseball, and basketball. Shane seemed genuinely interested in who I was and what had happened. While I didn't always trust displays of concern from other medical professionals, they felt real with Shane.

My dad took me to the movies afterward to reward me for keeping up with my therapy appointments. I liked spending time with him, and I had always liked movies. I didn't want to show my face (or rather have it be seen) in public, but the movies were somewhere I could relax a little bit. During the day, they were less busy than usual. Movies were dark and gave me a brief escape from reality. Even in the dark, I glanced around self-consciously to make sure no one was looking my way.

Because all of this took place in the winter, I tried to adapt to the challenge of walking on icy roads. I would slip and falter despite my best efforts. I didn't want to do any more damage to myself or be looked at by strangers with pity.

January days were short, bringing darkness even before dinnertime, which didn't help with my mental health. Seasonal Affective Disorder (SAD) is a real thing, let me tell you. I have always felt symptoms of it to a certain extent, but in combination with Ramsay Hunt syndrome, it had a big effect on me.

Even if I had a good day here or there and felt a small spark of hope for the future, it was never long before something would send me back down the spiral.

Because the extent of damage from Ramsay Hunt syndrome was still not fully known, I had to have my hearing tested.

The audiologist confirmed that I have permanent tinnitus and hearing loss. Yet one more limitation, one more thing to grieve.

I was taken to a balance testing centre where they put me through a series of tests. I had water put into my ear and was prompted to follow a red light with my eyes as the light moved from left to right.

At the end of the appointment, the doctor looked at me and sighed: "What are we going to do with you?"

I guess he'd never seen anyone with the extent of symptoms and damage I had, all in one patient, all in one appointment.

I stared furiously at my feet and tried not to lose it entirely. When I got home, I returned to my bedroom and the darkness where I could attempt to disappear.

At yet another appointment a couple of weeks later, I met with a nerve specialist. She looked at my chart, then at me. "There's a possibility that we can do facial nerve regeneration surgery."

No one else had mentioned surgery as an option until that day.

"We would take nerves from your leg and put them into your face, into the very canals where the affected nerves are no longer working so they can repair and regenerate."

Repair.

Regenerate.

I like those words.

"I have to warn you, though. It could take twelve to twenty-four months for the nerves to do anything of the sort."

I didn't care. It was something to reach for in the dark sea I was currently drowning in.

"Yes. I want to do surgery," I said immediately, jumping on any chance for "normality."

"Let's see how you do over the next two or three months and go from there."

I left that appointment feeling hopeful that when I saw her next, she would tell me I could have the surgery and "fix my face." I would have agreed to ten surgeries if that's what it took to be able to smile, close my left eyelid (I was wearing a patch to protect my eye from the elements by that point), and speak without struggle.

CHAPTER 3

DROWNING

Other than therapy appointments with Shane and movies with Dad, I'd given up everything and everyone I cared about before Ramsay Hunt changed my life. My mental health had deteriorated lower than I'd ever experienced in my life. In general, I'd always considered myself to be a strong guy, capable of handling what came my way. But this was no longer me. The only thing that kept me going at all was the potential for nerve surgery.

People encouraged me to have hope, cheer up, accept my new normal, fight harder, and be a warrior, but I didn't feel like much of a warrior at all. Instead, I was losing on all fronts.

One February afternoon, after waking up from a nap, I was at my mom's, waging my familiar daily battle with nausea and vertigo. My destination was the bathroom at the end of the hall. I *refused* to throw up in my bedside garbage pail again. The bathroom was only ten feet away, but it may as well have been ten miles. I held onto the wall with one hand and leaned on my cane with the other.

Just put one foot in front of the other, I told myself, trying not to lose patience. Shane would have been proud. There was a penalty to pay if I rushed—either a humiliating tumble to the floor or a brutal face-to-wood meetup with the guest bedroom's door frame.

Steady now . . . Five feet now . . .

I was just about past the hallway mirror when I caught a glimpse of my reflection with my good eye. As a rule, I tried to avoid all mirrors, but there was always that hopeful voice that asked, "What if the face I used to appreciate had abruptly returned to normal in my sleep?"

I knew better, yet sometimes, I just had to check. If my face could go askew while I was sleeping, who was to say it couldn't repair itself while I was sleeping?

Reality, that's who.

Then, all of this would be over, and I could go back to my life. I turned slowly to minimize the spin, faced the mirror as best as I could, and took in the reflection I had recently come to hate.

It was still broken, of course. It was asymmetrical as if someone had turned off the electricity to one side of my body. My left eye and my mouth still drooped down awkwardly.

I swore under my breath, turned too fast, lost my balance,

fell against the opposite wall and threw up on my mother's hardwood floors.

* * *

With the turn of April, we could all smell spring in the air. Usually, that was a relief, marking the long winter coming to an end. This year, it was a reminder that I should have been gearing up to start my paddleboarding season, which usually began mid-May.

Instead of getting back to business, I posted an announcement on social media and by email to announce that my business was closed. It took over an hour to press the send button and the second I did, I felt my heart break. Everything I'd created—everything I'd built—was gone.

I'd found great joy in working towards creating something that fulfilled me and brought joy to others. Now, what could I do?

Without purpose, it was a fight to keep my head above water. I slept late, I went to bed early, and I barely ate. I was a shell of my former self and not proud of it.

To the few people who I did let in, I was unrecognizable. I could see them trying to mask their shock and dismay. And failing.

The one thing that kept me going was knowing I had two vital medical appointments coming up.

On April 2, I went to the first one. It was with an otolaryngologist[8] (an ENT specialist) to see what could be done about my daily symptoms and their potential for improvement.

Dad sat beside me in the cold, sterile room that smelled of antiseptic. At least there was a window to let in some warmth and light.

The ENT came in and pulled my records up on his computer. I noticed he was handsome. He had a full head of hair and blue eyes.

"How are you doing?" he asked, without any warmth to match the light pouring in through the window.

I was truthful. "I've been doing vestibular rehab therapy, but it's not working the way I had hoped."

"Well, Ramsay Hunt syndrome has changed a lot of things with your nerves and brain chemistry," he explained, looking at my face. "And it will continue to."

Wait. I thought about his choice of words and felt my hands shake. Did that mean things would get worse? We were there for news on improvement, not decline!

As if to answer my darkest thoughts, he said, "Your capabilities are *different* now. We need to think about learning to live and adapt to those changes. Long car trips will make you dizzy

---

8   Clinic, Cleveland. 2023. "Otolaryngologist: What They Do & When to See One." Cleveland Clinic. January 23, 2023. https://my.clevelandclinic.org/health/articles/24635-otolaryngologist.

and sick. They are not advisable. Flying on airplanes is done. And your paddleboarding is done."

The way he so easily listed off the ways my life was over, as if reading from his grocery list, took my breath away.

Eggs? *Check.*

Bread? *Check.*

Career over? *Check.*

Life as you know it over? *Check.*

My dad led me out of that appointment, straight to the car, and that's where I broke down. As he drove us away from that awful office I hoped never to see again, I rested on the cold glass window. The despair I felt sucked up every ounce of energy I had. I couldn't bring myself to lift my head or sit up. I wanted to dissolve. I stared at the passing streets and buildings through tears, trying to hide them from my father, knowing I was failing badly.

"That guy was a piece of shit!" Dad growled, thumping his hand on the steering wheel. He was furious that the specialist had been so blunt without consideration for the life-altering declarations he was making and how they would affect the patient in front of him.

Two days later, we had a follow-up appointment with the nerve specialist about the possibility of having a facial nerve transplant. I was still shell-shocked from the ENT appointment and hanging on to Dad for dear life.

"Unfortunately, based on what we're seeing in your progress

and your MRIs, you are unfortunately not a viable candidate for the facial nerve transplant at this time."

So that was it. The ENT confirmed I would be unbalanced, nauseous, dizzy, and feeling horribly ill every day of my life. And now, the nerve specialist was saying that my facial paralysis would also never improve. *This* was the new me.

In two days, any hopes I had dared to hold out for were destroyed.

When we got outside the building, I broke down in tears in the parking lot. I was exhausted—from the pain, the isolation, the defeat, and the failure to see any improvement. My last glimmer of hope had been extinguished.

* * *

If I'd been treading water before, I wasn't anymore. This was drowning. I could feel, with every ounce of my being, that I was *done*. And yet, I was so wrong.

Today, I would give anything to go back to that day and tell myself how wonderful and full of purpose my life would become.

"It gets better" are the most magical, truthful words anyone could ever share or receive. But you have to be able or willing to hear them.

On that day, I couldn't see through the darkness in front of me. I had lost sight of hope.

That evening, I went online in search of any person willing

to sell me drugs. *A lot* of drugs. I knew that if I were going to have the courage to go through with this irreversible action, I would need to be so high, I was out of my mind.

I wrote a note to my mom, placed it in my underwear drawer and made my way downstairs.

"I'm going to a friend's place for the night," I told my mom as the taxi pulled up in front of the house.

"Really? That's great!" She was surprised because I didn't really do things like that anymore. I felt a sharp pang of guilt at the sound of her happiness.

"We're going to have pizza and watch movies. I will be back tomorrow," I said, knowing full well I wouldn't be coming back.

She looked me up and down, obviously taking note of my clothes and hair. I'd made an effort with my appearance, taking time to do my hair and dress the way I used to before RHS. It had taken hours because of how sick I was.

I knew I needed to look good, or at least "normal," to do what I had planned. I was worried that if I looked disabled, the person wouldn't sell me drugs.

"You look great!"

"Thanks, Mom. Love you." I hugged her, left the house, and made my way two hours away from home to the house of a stranger where I would be "safe" to spend hours getting high enough to go through with my plan.

The evening concluded with me attempting to take my life.

***

That evening was a blur, replayed only in short, sad movie trailers I wish I could forget. I remember an ambulance being called and police showing up as well. They were all alarmed by my fallen face and inability to walk. They must have thought it was from the drugs I had taken.

In my bed in the ER, people came in and out of my room. A heart monitor was hooked up to me. The nurses were concerned with how I presented. I told them about Ramsay Hunt and the symptoms and disabilities that had taken over my daily life. They listened with kindness and concern.

After telling my story, I mostly remained quiet. I was terrified they would admit me and put me in a padded room.

I'll never forget the wave of relief I felt when I heard the words, "You can go."

No psych ward, no straight jacket. My mental health crisis was camouflaged by my disabilities and drugs.

I took a cab to my dad's home where I woke up everyone in the house by banging on the door. When he answered, he could immediately tell I was high. He was angry that I was at his house, stoned and sloppy, where his wife and two young girls were asleep. He didn't want them to see me like that.

"Go lay down in the guest room," he said and went back to bed.

I did what I was told, curling up on the bed in a room

where I'd spent every other week for months. But this time, it felt very different. I couldn't sleep because of the drugs in my system.

The next evening, he took me to my mom's house. I was *still* high. I didn't know that was even possible. We barely talked on the way over. When we arrived, we went into her living room and all sat down.

I didn't know what to say. I couldn't stop shaking.

"Tell us what's going on, Mike," my dad said.

It took forever to find the words to start with, but then I did. I told them everything. The words wouldn't stop pouring out once they started. The dam was breaking.

"I hate who I am and what I've become. I hate how I don't see any possible way out. I am done. I don't want to be here anymore. I can't do it . . ." I talked about how the symptoms made me feel, how I hated the way people looked at me, how I hated feeling isolated, but then when people reached out and expressed pity, I hated that too.

When I was done, I felt a little bit better, as if I'd rid myself of toxic waste.

Mom and Dad both had tears in their eyes.

"This is not the way," Dad said. "If you continue down this path, you will die."

"I feel so alone. Even though you both do so much, I always feel so alone. I just can't go on like this anymore."

Mom put her hand on mine. "Mike, we love you."

"You need to get help with processing everything you've been through," my dad suggested, rubbing my back as I sobbed.

I could feel their heartbreak, and I hated myself for being the cause of it. But I could also feel their love. And that was one of the few things that meant anything to me by that point.

"I feel like I am a burden," I confessed. I didn't realize it, but this is a common emotion for people who are struggling with their mental health.

"You're not a burden. You just need some help," Dad said. "Will you let me take you for help?"

Being locked up, put in a straight jacket or a padded cell, or any of the versions of psychiatric wards I had heard of or seen on television, was one of my own personal nightmares. I shuddered in shame.

"You need help," Mom repeated.

I had no fight left in me. If there was a way to help me out of this feeling or help unbreak my parents' hearts, I'd do it.

"Okay," I whispered hoarsely.

CHAPTER 4

THE COMEBACK | FIRST STEPS

I packed a small bag with essentials, clothes, and a few personal items. I was scared, mostly of what I didn't know. What would a mental health facility be like? Padded room? Locked doors? I knew the facility I was going to was also one where people went when ordered to be there by the court.

I would be committing myself, which meant I was agreeing to stay there until doctors deemed me well enough to go back home.

I guess that meant I was surrendering.

I was scared that walking with a cane and wearing my pirate eye patch would make me even more vulnerable.

My dad and I barely spoke on the drive over. When we got there, he helped me with my bag but then turned around, got in his car, and drove away.

I'm alone. The thought sent a shiver down my spine.

I rang the doorbell. A voice came over the security intercom system and said, "Hi, Mike."

They were expecting me.

The door unlocked and opened at the sound of a buzzer. I stepped inside cautiously, unsure of what lay ahead of me.

I was now a patient at a mental health treatment facility.

* * *

I expected this place to be cold and hostile—an institution designed to strip you of your dignity and identity, a sterile place filled with faceless doctors and nurses who would see me as just another broken mind to be repaired.

But it wasn't that way at all. The warmth surprised me. It wasn't physical warmth; it was the kindness in the staff's eyes, the quietness in their voices. I wasn't expecting that.

The woman at the front desk smiled softly and handed me a bundle of clothes—a grey sweatshirt, sweatpants, and socks—and informed me that my own clothes would be washed.

"It's in case of bed bugs," she explained, though I suspected it was more about stripping away any remnants of the outside world. The clothes they gave me were soft and warm, but they weren't mine.

After the clothing switch, it was time for the intake. I sat in a small room across from a woman with piercing eyes. We went over my medications, my medical history, and—because they always ask this—the reason I was there. I muttered something about "needing help" but didn't elaborate. Did she want the story? Did I even want to tell it?

The rules and regulations were simple: stay safe, don't hurt myself, don't hurt anyone else, and we'd all get along.

They showed me to my room, and to my surprise, it was mine alone. Others had to share, but I'd lucked out—if you could call it that. The room was basic: a single bed, a dresser, and a nightstand with a lamp. It was ... fine.

I closed the door behind me, took a deep breath, and sat on the bed. I was thin from months of being sick, but the bed still creaked under my weight.

I don't know how many hours I stared at the wall in front of me that first day, trying to wrap my head around how I had ended up there.

The next day, my clothes were returned to me, washed and neatly folded. Putting them on made me feel a little more like myself.

I spent most of the next few days alone, holed up in that small room. Even though I had the freedom to wander, I didn't.

Room checks were frequent—staff popped in to check on me and others.

When I did occasionally leave my room or catch glimpses of other patients as they passed mine, I saw that some of them seemed to have a level of peace (they must have been here for a while), whereas others had sad, hollow eyes (likely lost in their own version of emotional hell). In one way or another, we were all struggling here. But we were safe.

* * *

There was a lot of time to fill. I didn't know how to be alone with my thoughts. The stillness became uncomfortable. It amplified the dark thoughts that ran on a never-ending loop.

I began to think about the people that came before me. How did others do it? How did they get through this? How long until things got easier? How many people had been through some version of this? I wasn't the first and certainly wouldn't be the last.

I started researching online, filling my time by finding answers. I wanted to understand the bigger picture. Before I knew it, I was deep into the history of mental health treatment in Canada. I poured over every bit of information I could find. The history of mental illness proved to be both horrifying and strangely comforting—and much of it made my own experience here feel small and insignificant in comparison.

In 1714, the treatment of the "mentally ill" in New France and British North America was up to the patient's family to deal with. A mental health ward was opened up in Quebec at the Hôtel-Dieu. Those who didn't have access to it and who couldn't be cared for at home would often end up in jail or poor houses. Conditions were overcrowded, unsanitary, and often had little food and no heat, no intervention, or treatment. There was also no medication, no therapy, and no understanding. People weren't seen as sick; they were seen as morally unfit. They were treated as sinners.

By the early 1800s, asylums were opened across Canada—places in name only. The first one was in Saint John, New Brunswick, in 1835, followed by another in Toronto a few years later. Some asylums were converted from abandoned jails. The one in Toronto had even started inside an abandoned jail before it moved into a wing of the Parliament Buildings.

What they received wasn't care; it was containment—patients strapped down and sedated with alcohol to keep them quiet.

Here I was, receiving support, with the freedom to move about, and staff who came in to check on me—not to lock me up or sedate me.

I tried to picture the people who had come through those early asylums. They must have been terrified.

The more I read, the more I realized just how much progress had been made.

***

Changes in care in Canada and the US were initiated by Dorothea L. Dix (1802–1887), Richard M. Bucke, Charles

K. Clarke, Clifford W. Beers (1876–1943) and Clarence M. Hincks (1885–1964).

Dorothea Dix was an American schoolteacher who had seen the horrors of these institutions firsthand. She travelled across Canada and the United States, exposing the deplorable conditions in which people were being kept. Because of her work, new hospitals were built—places where the mentally ill were treated with some degree of dignity. She also helped oversee the building of a hospital in Nova Scotia in the 1880s.

Dr. Richard Bucke became the superintendent of the "Asylum for the Insane" in Ontario—first in Hamilton in 1876, then in London a year later. He saw mental illness differently than most. To him, it wasn't a moral failing; it was part of the biological process of adapting to change. Bucke got rid of the alcohol they used to sedate patients, stopped restraining people, opened up spaces for cultural and sports events, and tried to create an environment where patients could actually heal.

Dr. Charles Clarke worked in the Hamilton asylum and later in Kingston. By the 1890s, Clarke had started advocating for the term *asylum* to be dropped entirely.

Clifford Beers was a Yale student who had a mental breakdown and ended up in an institution. He was abused, mistreated, and left to suffer. Despite all of that, he recovered and was released, which was when he wrote a book about his experience called *A Mind That Found Itself*. It became the foundation for the mental health movement in North America. Because of the firsthand account he was able to give of his own suffering and those of the other patients he witnessed in the asylum, people started to care. That's when real reform began.

Dr Clarence Hincks's interest in mental health was partly the result of his own experiences with severe depression. In 1918, with Beers's help, he organized the Canadian National Committee for Mental Hygiene, which later became the Canadian Mental Health Association. Hincks was one of the first physicians to recognize the value of prevention and treatment of sufferers of mental illness before they were incapacitated, which led to the development of child guidance clinics for the early detection and prevention of mental illness.[9]

* * *

There was a routine for everything at the facility which I found comfort in. After I'd researched just about everything I could, I was back to the silence. I knew I would eventually have to step outside myself and my little room if I were to have any chance of healing.

I wandered into the gated courtyard. The sun was out, and it felt good on my skin. I tried to focus on that to quiet my mind.

Later that day, I had my first session—a small group of

---

9   Goodman, John T.. "Mental Health." The Canadian Encyclopedia. Historica Canada. Article published February 07, 2006; Last Edited January 28, 2014.

us sat in a circle. I had no intention of spilling my darkest thoughts and feelings to a circle of strangers, so I crossed my arms, burned a hole through my running shoes with my gaze, and listened. One by one, others shared something. Listening to them slowed my racing heart, beat by beat, until when it came to my turn, something broke open. Words spilled out before I could stop them.

"I feel like a burden." My hands trembled in my lap. I spoke about my parents, about how they had become my caretakers—how I didn't want them to be. How I'd lost everything I thought I knew about myself. I admitted to how empty I felt. How hopeless.

And I cried. Harder than I had since it all began. The tears came without permission, but I didn't try to hide them this time.

That evening, something inside of me changed. I don't know what, but I found myself sitting in the dining area for dinner, eating with the others for the first time. I didn't feel hungry, but I forced the food down. Across from me sat a man named Rob. He looked rough—tattoos snaking up his arms and neck, the kind of person who'd make you cross the street if you saw him at night. But he wasn't what he seemed.

He spoke softly, asked about me, and listened without judgment. Turns out he was court-ordered to be there. He wasn't scary; he was kind and gentle. We talked. Then we watched a hockey game on the common room TV. For the first time since I'd arrived, I felt like I had someone—a friend.

In the days that followed, I opened up more than I had in the past six months. I started talking to the counsellors, unloading everything I'd kept inside. I was honest in a way I hadn't been with anyone, even myself. The staff became familiar faces, people I looked forward to seeing during their shifts. My initial fear of this place melted away. It wasn't the prison I thought it would be. It wasn't some torturous institution designed to break me down further. It was a place that, in its strange way, was beginning to heal me.

The others weren't what I had feared, either. They were simply—and hopefully temporarily—broken, just like me. I saw them for what they were—people. Just people struggling with an illness that, for many, was invisible.

* * *

Eventually, it was time to go home. I was put on mood stabilizers, which felt like admitting defeat at first, but I quickly learned to appreciate the way they made life feel less jagged. I had regular therapy appointments set up with both a psychologist and a counsellor.

The medication took time to work, but little by little, I noticed the change. At first, it was small—a lighter feeling in my chest, a tiny flicker of hope. My thoughts weren't as dark as they used to be. Therapy, too, began to help in ways I hadn't expected. Having someone to talk to, someone to really listen, made the difference. Despite my friends and family always offering to listen, I felt the weight of masking fall away. With counsellors, I didn't have to hide anything for fear of causing them worry.

It was strange to look forward to those appointments, to sit down with my counsellor in a coffee shop, updating her on how I was doing and how I was feeling. Slowly, I began to let go of the guilt, the shame of being a burden to my family. I learned to forgive myself.

I started looking forward to vestibular rehab appointments. It was another thing to put on my calendar, another place to go, another person to see—it was grounding.

* * *

One day in May, I received an email from the Canadian Safe Boating Council. They wanted me to do a presentation—something I had done every year before Ramsay Hunt. I stared at the screen, my heart pounding. *How could I stand in front of people when I couldn't even stand on my own? How could I demonstrate paddleboarding when I could barely walk without a cane?*

I closed the laptop, unwilling to face the request.

That evening, I mentioned it to a friend who owned a paddleboarding business. I asked her if she'd take my place. I would attend, but she would do the presentation. I liked the idea of passing the torch to her. It felt like the right thing to do.

When the day of the event came, I stood on the shore, cane in hand, watching from the sidelines. The media vans, the familiar faces, the warm sun—everything about that day felt surreal. I should've felt sad, but I didn't. Not really. I was just happy to be there.

When the demonstrations for the journalists and media crews wrapped up, it was just me and my friends—people I'd spent countless hours with on the lake in the past—remaining by the water. We were chatting and joking around. The boards were still floating, bobbing gently with the ripples of the lake.

"You wanna try, Mike?" asked one of them.

"No!" I snapped before I could stop myself. My confidence immediately disappeared, and I was almost angry that this was being suggested, ruining a nice morning.

I immediately wished I hadn't come. I just wanted to go home.

Someone said, "Try it for a few minutes and just see."

To my surprise, I heard myself agree, "Okay, we can try."

I put my cane on the grass, got strapped to a board, and put a life jacket on.

What the hell am I doing?! Is this even safe?

I envisioned myself moving my head too much or too fast, my vertigo making the world spin, and then falling off or, worse, drowning.

My head spun and my stomach somersaulted on the board, but I tried to focus on the water in front of me; all the while, my friends talked me through three of the longest minutes I've ever spent on the water. When the sun hit the surface of the lake and reflected onto my face, its warmth touched a part of myself that I forgot existed.

As I stepped back onto the sand, I could feel everyone's eyes on me, and even though I felt self-conscious and awkward, I also felt immediately hungry to try again.

From that moment forward, the water was my escape and my therapy. Over the summer, I spent more and more time on the board, pushing myself a little further each time.

My family and counsellors saw a change in me as pieces of my former self slowly returned. Shane noticed me getting stronger over the course of the summer. My sessions with him started to include me telling stories of being out on the water for five minutes one week, then ten the next. I hesitantly admitted how much joy and hope it brought me to gradually increase my time on the water with friends.

By mid-summer, something happened that I had thought impossible. I accidentally caught a glance of myself in the bathroom mirror, and at first, I didn't recognize myself.

I was used to bracing myself for the sight of my unevenness, the sag of my left cheek, the lopsided mouth . . . But this time was different.

I leaned in, close enough to see the faint lines around my eyes, the way my mouth twitched ever so slightly. The left side of my face, the one that had hung lifelessly for months, was starting to lift. The muscles were responding, pulling the skin back into place in a way they hadn't before. It wasn't perfect—it was still uneven—but there was a difference.

I saw it.

I *felt* it.

I blinked, trying to make sense of what I was seeing. My fingers reached up, almost unconsciously, tracing the side of my face. My skin felt warm, the same as it always had, but the movement beneath it—there was life there again. The muscles were working, fighting to bring back the symmetry I had lost. It was small and nearly imperceptible, but it was progress.

I tried to smile just a little, testing it out. My reflection smiled back—lopsided, yes, but more me than it had been in months. The left side lifted higher than it had before, not perfect, not yet, but trying.

Still me. But more familiar.

My body was still trying to heal. I wasn't sure how much longer it would take, but I wasn't frozen in time anymore. I was moving forward.

I stepped back from the mirror. There was no one around, no one to see my quiet, private victory. I almost wanted to tell someone, to share it, but I couldn't find the words.

I walked back to my room, the reflection still lingering in my mind. The unevenness was still there, but I saw something else now. *Progress. Possibility. A different future.*

* * *

Like a ripple effect, each tiny improvement led to another and another until, in late August, I was invited to share my story on stage in front of three hundred strangers. The idea of it terrified me. Three hundred people . . . looking at me . . . seeing me as I was . . . listening to *my* story.

My hands shook when I read the email. It felt wrong. Who was I to stand on a stage and talk about my journey when I still didn't fully understand it myself?

My mom and dad wanted me to do the talk. They were overflowing with support and encouragement. My friends also tried their best to convince me by promising to be there if I took the stage. In some way, the promise of their presence became a source of strength for me.

I threw myself into preparing for the talk. Hundreds of hours were spent memorizing, rehearsing, visualizing—trying to figure out how to tell my story in a way that would have a positive effect on others.

I wanted the audience to hear me, understand me, and maybe even laugh with me a little. I wanted them to feel entertained, to find something in my words that they could relate to. And when the day came, I stood there on that stage and told them everything.

I spoke about my mental health breakdown, about how the world had crumbled beneath me, and how, somehow, I had found my way back onto a paddleboard—the very thing I thought I'd lost forever.

I likened it to riding a horse, the way you get thrown off and have to decide whether to climb back on. I told them that we all go through that at different points in our lives—those moments where you hit the ground hard and have to figure out if you're brave enough to stand up again.

As I spoke, I felt the fear melting away. The audience wasn't just a crowd of strangers anymore. They were with me, listening, nodding, feeling what I felt.

By the time I finished speaking and took in the faces looking up at me, I realized they were standing now, giving me a loud, tearful, unexpected standing ovation. Something about my story had resonated with them in ways I had never imagined.

The talk was recorded, and when it was released online, it went viral, gaining millions of views across multiple online platforms and connecting me with strangers around the world.

People I'd never met were reaching out, sharing their own struggles, their own stories of getting knocked down and trying to get back up again. It was overwhelming, but in the best way. It showed me that I wasn't alone in feeling alone. There were others out there, struggling just like I had been.

That experience led me to write my first in a series of articles on mental health for the *Toronto Sun*. I wanted to share my story, but more than that, I wanted to talk about the bigger picture—the need for compassion, empathy, and understanding when it comes to mental health. The article didn't come without its challenges, though. After I sent it to my family, some of them told me not to submit it. "Maybe we aren't there yet," they said. "Maybe it's too soon." They feared there may be consequences to sharing something so personal.

But I knew it needed to be out there. So, despite their reservations, I asked the editor to run it.

The article went to print, and not long after, *Healthing* picked it up and ran it nationally in every Postmedia newspaper across Canada. It felt surreal to see my words spread across the country, knowing so many people were reading about me. But more than that, it felt like the beginning of something bigger.

With each sharing of my story, I became braver, stronger. I had a sense of purpose. It had been so long since I'd felt that.

I wasn't just surviving anymore.

I was living. And that was everything.

CHAPTER 5

SPEAKING | INNOVATION

In March of 2020, the world came to a standstill. I remember the exact moment the gravity of it hit me. I was sitting in the greenroom of *Breakfast Television* at the Citytv building, waiting to go on air to promote facial palsy awareness week. As I nervously went over talking points in my head, trying to ignore my usual pre-interview jitters, my eyes drifted to a whiteboard hanging on the wall. There, hastily scrawled in black marker, was the count of COVID-19 cases in Canada. The numbers were small but rising fast. Other countries were in the tens of thousands of cases already.

That was the first time I stopped and asked myself, *How bad is this going to get?*

That week was significant for other reasons, too. Earlier in March, I had reconnected with an old college friend, Lisa, who worked in public affairs lobbying governments to create meaningful change. She was savvy, clever, and connected—everything you'd want in a public affairs professional. I had reached out to her to help me lobby the Ontario government to lower the age requirement for the shingles vaccine. Getting that vaccine could have prevented me from getting Ramsay Hunt syndrome. I didn't want anyone else to go through what I had endured.

Lisa took the idea and ran with it, setting up meetings with key political figures—everyone from the interim leader of the Liberals to officials in the Ontario Ministry of Health. Each meeting felt like a step forward, a tangible move toward real change. When I walked through the halls of the Ontario Legislature, I was filled with a kind of excitement I hadn't felt in a long time. This was where decisions were made, where laws were passed, and where change was born. And I was there to do something that mattered—not just for me, but for anyone who might face what I had.

But just three days after my *Breakfast Television* appearance, the world changed. I think it was when the NBA suspended all basketball games that it became clear—everything was about to change.

In the days that followed, the world unravelled. Fear crept into all of our lives. Fear of losing the people we loved. Fear of isolation, the unknown.

It was eerie. The streets emptied, as did the food shelves. Grocery stores became battlegrounds for toilet paper, masks, and hand sanitizer.

I was still living with my mom at the time, so I had a

support system. Together, we hunkered down like the rest of the world, watching as everything unfolded and grew worse than any of us had dared to imagine.

As the pandemic unfolded, conversations about vaccines dominated the headlines, but they weren't the vaccines I'd been fighting for. Suddenly, my battle to lower the age requirement for the shingles vaccine felt insignificant. Who would care about that now when the whole world was scrambling to develop a vaccine to prevent people from dying? The meetings I had fought for, the momentum we'd built—all of it dissolved overnight.

By summer, social media apps were filled with ominous videos of people walking down empty streets in some of the biggest cities in the world, including Toronto.

Work had become remote for nearly everyone. The city had fallen into the longest lockdown in all of North America. For my birthday that year, we tried to recreate some semblance of normalcy. We ordered steaks from a butcher and pretended we were dining out at The Keg, my favourite restaurant. We rented a movie, got snacks, and tried to make it feel like a night out at the theatre. It wasn't the same, of course, but there was something comforting in the attempt. It was a way of clinging to the familiar, even as everything else spun out of control.

The first time I cried during the pandemic took me by surprise. It happened after a grocery run. I was walking through the aisles, carefully maintaining my distance from everyone else, watching people follow stickers on the floor, shuffling around like zombies, their faces half-covered by masks.

Many people faked optimism (we're Canadians, after all), but their eyes were sad, anxious, and angry . . . I had seen those eyes before in the mental health facility when patients first checked in. I'd seen them in my own mirror on some of my darkest days.

It hit me how alone I felt. How alone we all were. I couldn't wait to get back home to my safe space, my regulations-approved "bubble" consisting of my mom and me.

This wasn't just a pandemic risking the physical health of everyone we knew and loved. It was a mental health crisis, too.

A DEEP DIVE INTO MENTAL HEALTH STATISTICS

In any given year, one in five Canadians experiences mental illness.[10] In fact, by the time Canadians reach forty years of age, one in two have – or have had – a mental illness.[11]

Major depression affects approximately 5.4 percent of the Canadian population with anxiety disorders close behind at 4.6 percent of the population.[12] About one percent of Canadians

---

10 Smetanin et al. (2011). The life and economic impact of major mental illnesses in Canada: 2011-2041. Prepared for the Mental Health Commission of Canada. Toronto: RiskAnalytica.
11 Smetanin et al., 2011
12 https://www.doi.org/10.25318/82-003-x202001200002-eng

will experience bipolar disorder (formerly called "manic depression"), and another one percent will experience schizophrenia.[13] Eating disorders affect approximately one million Canadians. They impact women at a rate ten times that of men and have the highest rate of mortality of any mental illness.[14] Substance use disorders affect approximately six percent of Canadians.[15]

About four thousand Canadians per year die by suicide. That's an average of almost eleven suicides per day.[16] It affects people of all ages, education, income levels, and cultures; however, systemic inequalities such as racism, poverty, homelessness, discrimination, colonial and gender-based violence, among others, can worsen mental health and symptoms of mental illness, especially if mental health supports are difficult to access.

In Canada, suicide disproportionately impacts Indigenous peoples; the rate of suicide among First Nations is three times higher than among non-Indigenous Canadians, and nine times higher among Inuit.[17] The mortality rate due to suicide among men is three times the rate among women, but girls and young

---

13 "Fast Facts about Mental Health and Mental Illness." 2021. CMHA National. November 17, 2021. https://cmha.ca/brochure/fast-facts-about-mental-illness/.
14 "Section D - Eating Disorders." 2012. Statcan.gc.ca. January 30, 2012. https://www150.statcan.gc.ca/n1/pub/82-619-m/2012004/sections/sectiond-eng.htm.
15 Mental Health Commission of Canada. n.d. "Making the Case for Investing in Mental Health in Canada." https://www.mentalhealthcommission.ca/wp-content/uploads/drupal/2016-06/Investing_in_Mental_Health_FINAL_Version_ENG.pdf.
16 Statistics Canada (2020). Deaths and age-specific mortality rates, by selected grouped causes. Table 13-10-0392-01
17 Canada,. 2016. "The Daily — Suicide among First Nations People, Métis and Inuit (2011-2016): Findings from the 2011 Canadian Census Health and Environment Cohort (CanCHEC)." Statcan.gc.ca. 2016. https://www150.statcan.gc.ca/n1/daily-quotidien/190628/dq190628c-eng.htm.

women are three times more likely than men to harm themselves and be hospitalized from self-harm.

No one is immune to mental health challenges. Some suffer more than others, but all of us will pay for it—in particular, employers.

A CBC report claims that stigma surrounding mental health costs employers $20 billion a year.

- Lack of access to mental health services and unfriendly environments to discuss mental health lead to absenteeism, lack of productivity, and rising claims among employees.
- Among a variety of workplaces, psychological problems make up seventy percent of disability costs.
- Workplace aside, mental health claims can cost the Canadian economy upwards of $50 billion according to the Mental Health Commission.[18]
- The stigma around mental illness remains a huge barrier to improving mental health in the workplace, a problem the Mental Health Commission of Canada estimates costs employers $20 billion a year. Mental health problems account for one in three workplace disability claims, the commission says, contributing

---

18 "The State of Mental Health in Canada - CCLA." 2017. CCLA. February 9, 2017. https://ccla.org/get-informed/talk-rights/the-state-of-mental-health-in-canada/?gad_source=1&gclid=Cj0KCQjwrKu2BhDkARIsAD7GBovEIcqhB0p5QRIuwp-WVH946X-hOPz2-ACDeb1-WElsIxxCf2wer48saAuAJEALw_wcB.

to absenteeism and lack of productivity as well as health costs.

- To put this another way, in any given week, five hundred thousand Canadians may miss work because of mental illness. Different workplaces have different problems—high absenteeism among health-care workers, post-traumatic stress among first responders, substance-abuse problems among oil and gas workers—but almost seventy percent of disability costs were related to psychological problems.[19]

* * *

As the months dragged on, the pandemic's mental health impact was impossible to ignore. Every conversation revolved around isolation and loneliness. People were struggling, parents were worried about their kids, and there was a shared sense of hopelessness that hung in the air. One conversation in particular stuck with me. I was talking to my friend Andrea about her daughter's experience—how hard it had been for her to be separated from her friends, how much she missed her old routines. Listening to her, I tried to imagine this situation through the eyes of a child.

---

19   "Stigma around Mental Illness a $20B Problem in Workplace." 2015. CBC. November 3, 2015. https://www.cbc.ca/news/business/mental-illness-workplace-1.3295242.

I had isolated myself during my own mental health struggles, so in a strange way, I felt like I had already been through this—like I had been training for these moments, my own personal Olympics.

The resilience I had built during my recovery was now serving me well, but I knew that wasn't the case for millions of others around the world. People were breaking under the pressure of isolation, and it reminded me once again how crucial mental health support was, especially for younger people.

In June, amid the chaos, I decided we would still move forward with my annual paddleboarding event to support Jack.org, a national nonprofit that provides mental health programs for youth and Canada's largest network of young leaders transforming the way young Canadians think about mental health. I had connected with them right after the time my talk went viral, asking them how I could help.

The event had always been a way to bring people together, to raise awareness and support for a cause now close to my heart. But this time, it felt different. We had to scale back—fewer participants, more restrictions, and the looming fear of another lockdown. I had hoped for hundreds of people, but we barely reached a hundred.

I was disappointed, of course. When you organize events, you always want to build on the success of the previous year, to grow, to reach more people. But the world wasn't the same, and neither was the event. As people left that day, I felt an odd sense of finality. I wished I had stayed longer, talked to more people, and soaked it all in. I didn't realize it at the time, but that would be the last time we held that event.

Days later, Toronto went back into lockdown. The longest lockdown in North America. And just like that, we were all back in our homes, disconnected from each other once again.

By November, I was on a call with Jack.org, discussing the annual event and admitting how disappointed I was. The pandemic had stripped away so much of what I had hoped to achieve, but everything was on hold indefinitely. As the news ticker flashed frightening numbers of cases and deaths across the screen, I knew we couldn't plan for another event next year. It was too uncertain, too risky. And so, we made the hard decision not to move forward.

I hung up the phone, feeling defeated.

* * *

Like in many houses across the world, news was on the TV at some point each day. One night, a story popped up about Marilyn Bell—the youngest person to swim across Lake Ontario back in 1954. She had swum fifty kilometres from New York to Toronto, becoming a national hero. The story stuck with me, looping in my mind like a broken record.

A few days later, I called Jack.org with a new idea.

* * *

I was invigorated for the first time in months. We couldn't gather in groups, but what if we could build something different?

What if I tried to paddleboard across Lake Ontario?

> LAKE ONTARIO has the last smallest surface area (19,000 square kilometres) of the Great Lakes. It is fed by the Niagara River at the bottom of Niagara Falls, and flows to the Atlantic Ocean via the St. Lawrence River. As the final lake in the Great Lakes chain, it is both the lowest in mean surface elevation and the worst in water pollution levels of all the Great Lakes.[20]

The idea felt wild at first, but the more I thought about it, the more it made sense. We couldn't plan traditional events, but we could still raise awareness for the mental health crisis.

The idea had been rattling around in my head for days, like a puzzle piece that just wouldn't fit until suddenly, it clicked. It felt almost absurd—trying to pull off something this big in the middle of a global pandemic—but it was exactly the kind of boldness I needed.

We couldn't gather in close proximity. We couldn't hold

---

20 Wikipedia Contributors. 2024. "Lake Ontario." Wikipedia. Wikimedia Foundation. October 6, 2024. https://en.wikipedia.org/wiki/Lake_Ontario.

our traditional events. But we could create something different. Something people could cheer for from a distance. Something they could watch unfold and feel connected to, even while separated by miles and screens.

I could see the hesitation in the team at Jack.org when I brought it up on our next call. They weren't expecting this. I wasn't even sure I had expected it, but once I'd spoken the words, I couldn't take them back. They were out there now, like the spark of a match.

The goal was to raise awareness and funding for Jack.org.

I wanted to show and inspire people to believe that no matter how dark things got, there was always a way forward.

I reassured the Jack.org team: I would train, I would build a team, I was physically well enough to attempt this, it wasn't a spur-of-the-moment decision; I had been thinking about it, turning it over and over in my mind, imagining what it would take to make it happen. And now, I was ready. My mind was clear, my body stronger than it had been in years, and I knew this was the challenge I needed. Not just for me, but for everyone who had been struggling through this pandemic. This wasn't just about me crossing the lake. It was about showing that even in the darkest times, we could still do something remarkable.

By the end of November, the team at Jack.org was on board. The initial hesitation had shifted into excitement, their voices filled with the kind of energy I had been craving since the world shut down. We weren't just planning an event; we were planning a story of resilience and hope. I knew the crossing wouldn't be easy. It would take months of preparation, training, and overcoming countless obstacles. But we all agreed—this was worth it.

By the time we wrapped up the call, we had set our sights on August of the following year. In just nine months, I would attempt to paddle across Lake Ontario.

As I hung up, I felt a rush of adrenaline, the kind I hadn't felt in so long. For the first time in months, I had something to look forward to. A purpose. A goal that pushed me beyond the walls of isolation, back into the world, even if only figuratively at first.

I stared out of the window, the early winter light casting long shadows across the backyard. The leaves had long since fallen, and the grass was starting to fade beneath the chill of November. But all I could see was August—the open water, the horizon stretching ahead, and me, pushing forward, paddle in hand. I could see it all, clear as day.

The world might have been locked down, but I'd found a way forward. This would be my crossing—not just of a lake, but of everything that had held me back.

I started sending out emails, reaching out to sponsors, planning logistics, and trying to bring this bigger-than-life idea into reality.

There were barriers, of course—hundreds of emails went unanswered at first. But I kept pushing. This project became my lifeline, something that gave me purpose again. Every time I worked on it, I felt a sense of excitement and hope.

As Christmas of 2020 approached, I couldn't help but feel a sense of gratitude. I thought back to how different everything had felt just two years earlier, entering the holiday season with the intention of it being my last.

But now, here I was, in my family bubble, not only alive but carrying news. *Big news.*

For days, I had been rehearsing how I would tell them about my plan to paddleboard across Lake Ontario.

Telling my parents was the hardest part. I was scared of their reactions, scared they might think I wasn't strong enough to pull this off, and scared of their arguments against me doing this. I prepared for the conversation like I was going into a debate, making a list of points to refute any objections they might have. I wanted them to approve. I needed their support.

But when the time came, there were no arguments. There was only love, support, and a level of belief in me that I hadn't expected.

My parents were all in.

***

As the new year began, I knew I had to take my news public. I took to social media and announced that in August, I would attempt to paddleboard from Rochester, New York, to Toronto, Ontario.

The response was overwhelmingly positive, further building my confidence that I could do this.

In the early winter months, training took a back seat to the campaign logistics—detailed planning, sponsors, and media coverage. Looking back, that was a mistake. I should have focused more on building my physical strength.

Every day, I'd wake up early and sit in front of my computer, reaching out to businesses, corporations, and anyone I could think of. It felt like I was reaching out to the entire world, asking for support.

Days turned into weeks and then into months. My life revolved around this. Sometimes, I spent sixteen hours a day on the computer, obsessively contacting people, pushing, and hoping for a breakthrough. My family and friends noticed the change before I did. They'd ask me to come out, to take a break, but I couldn't. I felt like I had to keep going, had to keep pushing through. After all, they say that for every yes you get, there are a hundred noes before it. And I needed a lot of yeses to make this work.

I kept going, enduring the rejection, determined to build a meaningful awareness campaign that would help as many people as possible.

But as time went on, I grew tired of rejection—or, in many cases, no replies at all. It was isolating. I couldn't understand why it was so hard to get people to care. Social media was flooded with stories of people struggling with their mental health during the pandemic—parents worried about their kids, families feeling the strain of isolation—so why weren't they jumping on board? Did they only care about their own struggles? I didn't have time to dwell on it. I had work to do.

*　*　*

I knew I needed a team. This wasn't something I could do alone. After extensive research, it was determined I would need two boat captains, three people with the ability to operate motorboats, and a six-person crew to handle logistics, navigation, and safety.

We pieced the team together in the final stages of the campaign, and it showed. The team felt disjointed, like two separate groups that never fully clicked, but they were all there to support me and the cause. Despite the friction, I was just grateful to have people who believed in the mission.

The date for crossing Lake Ontario from Rochester, New York, to Toronto was set for August 22, 2021, rain or shine.

It was February already, and I quickly realized I'd neglected something crucial: my training. I got back on the paddleboard for the first time in months.

I began making weekly trips to Lake Ontario, even in

freezing temperatures, working with my friend Sebastien. He owned a paddleboard business and did his best to help me build up my strength and endurance. Together, we'd paddle through icy waters, practicing laps and working on speed while manoeuvring through ice chunks.

By spring, I knew I needed to do more, so I started hitting the gym every day, desperate to make up for lost time.

In June, with the crossing date growing closer, I was thrust into the public eye again. The *Toronto Star* decided to run a two-page story on me for the Life Section, covering my journey from my fall to my rise and this big, ambitious attempt. It was the first real media attention the event had received around my goal to cross Lake Ontario. As it turned out, the coverage was invaluable, bringing eyes and attention to the organization receiving the benefits of our efforts.

The *Toronto Star* sent a photographer to take photos of me on Toronto Island to go with the article. Soon after, the story was everywhere. Television networks picked it up. CP24, CTV News, Global, CBC—they all wanted to feature the story. The attention came fast, and with it came a new kind of pressure. I remember going to the beach for an interview with CP24's *Breakfast Host* Bill Coulter, and they sent out a helicopter to get aerial shots of me on the water. I couldn't stop looking up at the helicopter, which triggered my vertigo, making me feel dizzy and nauseous the entire time.

That day, word spread through the Toronto beaches

neighbourhood about the helicopter and the guy who was going to paddle across Lake Ontario.

The buzz was building.

* * *

By August, the media attention was at its peak. Jack.org was thrilled with how much awareness the crossing campaign was bringing to their cause, and we hadn't even left the shore yet.

Their Jack.org annual bike ride (their primary awareness and fundraising event up to that point) involved hundreds of volunteers and usually garnered a handful of media hits. But the crossing was far exceeding their media expectations, and they were impressed.

But the attention took its toll on me.

With each interview and each appearance, I felt more and more physically drained. It wasn't long before that it would take hours just to get dressed and do my hair to leave the house. Being in the media, doing interviews, doing photoshoots, and training—essentially being "on" all the time as an ambassador for the organization and a spokesperson for mental health—was exhausting, especially with my neurological condition.

There were days when I simply couldn't keep up. I'd crash and spend twenty-four hours straight just sleeping to try to recharge for what was ahead.

The pressure to get the messaging right and represent Jack.org in the best possible light was overwhelming.

People closest to me began to notice a significant weight loss. Friends and family began to worry, commenting on how thin I'd become and how tired I looked. I had lost twenty pounds.

I was so consumed with the campaign that I often forgot to eat. I'd tell myself I'd grab something later, but "later" would turn into dinner, and sometimes dinner wouldn't happen at all. This wasn't just a few bad days. This had been the reality for months.

Even I could see it in the photos—the way my face had grown gaunt, the way I looked fragile, sickly. I was about to attempt something monumental and needed to be at the top of my game, but instead, I was going into it exhausted, burned out, and dangerously thin.

I knew, deep down, that I wasn't ready. I needed more time—another two or three months at least—but the date was set, and I felt like I had no choice but to push through.

After all, we'd agreed to a date, rain or shine.

That was a mistake.

* * *

We often celebrate people who are brave enough to talk about their failures. We highlight the lessons they've learned from their experiences, romanticizing the struggle, the pain, and the perseverance. But the truth is that failure is usually messy. Ugly even. It's raw and complicated, and it doesn't always come with a neatly packaged lesson tied up in a bow.

Failure is defined as the lack of success, the inability to meet an expectation. The problem is, we tend to read too much into it. We tie failure to our self-worth, to our identity. And too often, the expectation we fail to meet is our own—a bar we've set impossibly high in our own heads.

When I think about the crossing of Lake Ontario in 2021, I no longer view it as a regret. I can say that now, but at the time, even in the days leading up to the event, through the crossing itself and in the aftermath, regret consumed me. It ate away at me like a slow, persistent ache. I saw that attempt as a defining character trait—one that would either label me as a success or as a failure.

That was also a mistake.

* * *

The team for that crossing was the last thing I assembled. It should have been the first.

All I knew was that I was desperate for support. In the end, my support team consisted of seven people on two motorboats. One boat was captained by Rob, a former professor of mine from college, and his wife. The other boat didn't come together until six weeks before the crossing. A man named Keith and his wife Sarah, from Oshawa, Ontario, answered a call I had put out on social media requesting a boat and a captain.

Meeting Keith for the first time was a turning point. We met at Whitby Marina after exchanging a few text messages, and when I first saw him—a big guy with a solid build and a no-nonsense demeanour—I didn't know what to expect. But he turned out to be a kind man who immediately welcomed me and treated me like family. A journeyman for Ontario Power Generation, Keith's beard hid a big smile and a laugh that always put me at ease.

That first day, he greeted me with snacks and an invitation to take his boat out for a spin "to see if it would do," he said.

If it would do?

This man and his wife had offered up a fully decked-out motorboat, complete with cabins for sleeping, a kitchen, and bathrooms, and he was asking me *if it would do.*

I knew within moments of meeting Keith that I had made a new friend.

Over the next two weeks, I spent nearly every evening on the water with Keith. He followed me on his boat while I paddled to test how that would work in daylight and darkness. We went over logistics for the crossing—discussing routes, supplies, and team support. We spent hours going over the path from Rochester, New York, to Toronto, Ontario, figuring out where we could stop for food and where I could rest. Every night, as the sun set over the marina, I felt more and more confident. Keith believed in me, and that belief was something I hadn't felt from anyone outside of my family in a long time. It gave me the sense of safety and security I needed. I only wish the rest of the crossing team had instilled that same confidence in me.

* * *

Even though we said "rain or shine" for the crossing date of August 22, Keith and I set a backup day of August 23, just in case of bad weather. For the record, the weather often lasted more than one day, but it was my conciliation. Fortunately, the forecast looked clear—favourable winds, calm water. Everything was in place.

We transported coolers of food and supplies to the boats, and then, on August 21, two boats with two teams left for Rochester, the American side of the crossing. Rob's boat left from Belleville, Ontario, while Keith's departed from Oshawa. The plan was to dock overnight in Rochester, prepare everything for the morning, and start the crossing bright and early.

The boat ride to Rochester took about two and a half hours, travelling at top speed. Keith encouraged me to stay below deck in the sleeping cabins to rest, but my nerves were too fried. The excitement and anxiety made sleep impossible.

When we docked in Rochester, I finally emerged from below deck, greeted by the smell of snacks that Sarah had laid out. Her warmth and generosity, much like Keith's, slowed my racing heart. I focused on enjoying every bite, knowing that every calorie would be needed in the coming hours.

Keith and Sarah took turns driving the boat, supporting each other like they had done this a hundred times before. We joined up with Rob's boat, which had docked an hour earlier, and spent the rest of the afternoon walking around the marina, soaking in the sun before returning to the boat for a barbecue dinner.

It felt like the calm before the storm. Even though I was surrounded by chatter and camaraderie, inside, my mind was going over the events of the next day. I'd flash a smile whenever it felt like the right time, but inside, I was on another planet.

That night, after dinner, the team gathered to go over the final plan. We agreed on an 8:30 a.m. start, and I went to bed. I remember hearing voices below deck—serious voices—as I dozed off. Something in their tones told me something was wrong, but I'd hit my limit and crashed hard.

In the morning, I learned that a tropical storm had hit New Jersey and New York City overnight. *That must have been why everyone was sounding so serious.* It was moving up the eastern seaboard faster than expected, and we were now in a race against time. Despite what some people might think, most weather systems, especially storms that swept up the eastern seaboard, eventually landed in Canada and moved across our Great Lakes.

We were informed that it would be less than a day before the storm hit Lake Ontario.

There was no benefit in waiting a day. That would have made the situation and risk worse. So, we stuck with our original date.

I remember sitting at the end of the pier, watching the sun rise and paint the sky a brilliant red. I felt a strange sense of calm wash over me. For a moment, I didn't think of logistics, media, risk, strength, or danger. I only admired the beauty of it all. That is, until I remember what a red sky in the morning meant: *sailors take warning.*

I was about to cross a Great Lake that was nearly 244 metres deep, along a nearly 150 km path, on a paddleboard, through a storm.

***

I was dropped off at the main beach by the crew at 8 a.m. Two news teams were coming to interview me and cover the launch, and I was relieved they'd be there. Even though I knew my boats would be offshore waiting for me, I didn't want to start this alone.

As I prepared to launch, I was surprised by a visitor—Pat Labez, a woman from New York City who had driven all the way to Rochester to see me off. She hugged me like a mother, telling me how proud she was. She mentioned the storm and how difficult it had been to get out of the city because of the rain, which meant the storm was closer than I had hoped.

When I saw Keith's boat out on the water, I waded in up to my knees, climbed onto my board, and paddled out to meet them. When I reached the boat, Keith looked down from the helm and asked, "Are you ready?"

Am I ready?

I wasn't sure if anyone could ever really be ready for something like this. All I knew was that I had to take the first paddle if we were going to do this.

So, I did.

Eerily, the morning was calm. The weather held as we paddled west along the American shoreline, but the wind picked up as the day went on. The water grew choppier, harder to navigate. Every two hours, we stopped so I could eat and hydrate. Turkey sandwiches on plain bagels and Gatorade became my fuel, something to look forward to as the boat engines powered down and the world grew still, if only for a moment.

As the day wore on, the swells grew larger, and the waves hit harder. I found myself paddling faster while sitting down than standing up, the chop making it almost impossible to maintain balance. Rob, ever observant, realized I was motivated by being between the two boats. When I was behind them, I felt like I was falling short, so we adjusted the positioning to keep me centred between the two.

The American shoreline, dotted with trees, summerhouses, and sandy beaches, became my visual anchor as we pushed forward. But as the day turned into night, the real challenge began. The sky darkened, the water grew even more disorienting, and my team strapped lights to me so they could see me in the water.

Navigating the night was nothing like the day. I wasn't allowed to play music because I needed to be hyper-aware of the boats and the communication between us. The wind howled, and the waves continued to grow, throwing us off course.

My team began to feel the strain. Several crew members became violently seasick, and by the morning of the second day, exhaustion weighed heavy on everyone.

The breaks to feed me became increasingly more dangerous with the waves—and the paddleboard with me on it—pounding against the sides of the boats.

On the second day, as the sun came up, I felt a rush of energy. I was more motivated to conquer this lake than ever, fuelled by knowing we had come this far. Seeing our progress helped me stay focused on my goal.

Unfortunately, the morning weather intensified with wind gusts and waves. I watched as my support boats went up five-foot swells and then came crashing down, only to be lifted up once again, over and over.

The boats could no longer travel in a straight line, so they started zigzagging through the water to avoid hitting each other or me.

We stopped to feed me in the early afternoon, and I knew right away that something was wrong. The crew of Rob's boat called me over.

"Both of our teams are seasick," Rob said. "The weather isn't getting any better. It's time to call it. For everyone's safety, including yours."

I didn't know what to say. I was starving, and my muscles were screaming, but I wanted to keep going. I knew there was no point in voicing my objections; the decision had been made.

I was helped onto the boat by members of the team who assured me that it was for the best and there was no other way.

Captain Keith and the crew members on the other boat were updated by radio.

They decided to travel west and dock for the night on the American side. It was closer than attempting to cross the lake, which could've been potentially dangerous at that point.

I think I was in shock, either by physical exertion or by the executive decision to give up after so much planning and preparation.

"Why don't you go downstairs to rest," someone, I don't remember who, suggested.

I numbly nodded and went down to the cabin, shut the door, fell onto the bed, and sobbed. I couldn't have stopped it if I tried.

I had let everyone down—friends, family, the Jack.org team,

my teams, the media, the people suffering within the mental health crisis, myself . . . everyone.

When we finally arrived at the marina, there was tension in the air between the two teams. We had been divided by the decision to call it.

This is not the community I remembered from the night before we left Rochester, the ones who barbecued and laughed and dreamed big about what this crossing meant to the world.

Now, the two teams ate separately, and the atmosphere was one of anger and resentment.

After dinner, inside Captain Rob's boat, we started writing an announcement I would have to read to the media to explain my failure.

We spent two hours drafting a message focusing on how this was a success, reviewing the lessons we learned, and finishing off with a promise to be back.

No matter what the spin was, it felt like I was putting my failure in black and white.

I thought about the time and events that had led up to that moment and felt tormented over whether the team had made the right decision or not. I only knew that everything we'd worked for was done.

When everyone finally fell asleep, I slipped out of the boat and went for a walk in the middle of the night. I tried to process the events of the last two days. I forgot my shoes and was pacing in bare feet in our otherwise empty New York marina parking lot at 2 a.m. I was on the phone, panicking about what would happen the next day. *No one will understand.* It was a thought that ran on repeat for hours.

The following morning, we crossed the lake by boat. My team dropped me off on my paddleboard about fifteen kilometres out from shore so that I could paddle in and make the announcement in person to people waiting on shore.

When we got five kilometres from shore, the Toronto Marine Police Unit arrived with two officers who accompanied me the rest of the way. This let my support crews off the hook to go ahead of me, dock, and be there to meet me on shore when I arrived.

Even though I was distraught, the officers and I had a really nice conversation as we made our way to the Toronto beaches.

As I arrived, I was greeted by friends, family, supporters, the Jack.org organization, and reporters. I will never forget their cheers as I stepped off the board for the last time. I was completely overwhelmed with emotion, trying to wipe away my tears.

After a few hugs, I was guided to the microphones where I read the prepared statement. It was a struggle to stay composed and get through the words.

I was going through the prescribed motions, but I was not really there. In my mind, I was reliving the events out on the water and the weeks and months leading up to it, wondering what I could have done differently to prevent failure.

In my eyes, this was not just a failure of mind and body versus the elements; it was a failure of project management, team building, execution, and me. My confidence was shattered.

I was about to learn why some of the world's top leaders have catapulted themselves to the forefront of their industries on the backs of their own failures. Those are the leaders who learned the hard way that failure is the best teacher, a priceless (or expensive) learning opportunity that was worth every penny.

The media was already asking about when I'd try again. I was still in shock and not sure how to answer.

I still had a dream, but I now knew that the bigger the dream, the bigger the potential for failure. And I—along with my friends, supporters, and the organization—was learning that humbling lesson on live television in real time.

CHAPTER 6

LAKE ONTARIO | FAILURE

One of my favourite parts of living in Southern Ontario was getting to experience all four seasons. Fall has always been my favourite: warm days, cooler nights, the comfort of sweaters, and the smell of hot apple cider. It was a season that reminded me to slow down, take in the changes around me, and enjoy the quieter moments before winter's chill set in. I struggled to find comfort that year. A feeling of failure, defeat, and loss followed me throughout each day.

People said the crossing attempt was a success, but I didn't see it that way. Sure, I had paddled further than most would even consider, and I'd brought attention to the cause, but all I could focus on was that I didn't finish.

Wherever I went, someone wanted to talk about the crossing. I had shone a big, bright spotlight on the campaign, so it only made sense for it to be the topic of conversation.

Everyone wanted to know more. How did I feel? Would I try again next summer?

Each conversation was like picking at an open wound, but I didn't know how to make it stop.

There I was, surrounded by people who wanted to support me, and yet I felt deeply, profoundly alone.

On Thanksgiving weekend, I went to my dad and stepmom's house. The house was filled with smells of turkey, vegetables, and the sweet smells of baked desserts. The house and dinner table were decorated for the season. It was comforting. We all sat down for dinner as a family—me, my sisters, and my parents—and began exchanging stories about what was going on in our lives and what our plans for the winter were. And as the conversation unfolded, something gnawed at me.

I had no idea what my plans were. I needed to figure out what I was going to do. I needed to figure out what was coming next for me.

* * *

That night, back home, I pulled out some of the newspaper articles that had been written during the crossing attempt. I had saved them all, even though reading them felt like a double-edged sword. As I skimmed through the articles, one from the *Toronto Star* caught my eye. It mentioned Vicki Keith.

Vicki Keith was a Canadian retired marathon swimmer, a coach, and an advocate for disabled athletes. Her accomplishments were nothing short of extraordinary. She was the first and only person to swim across all five Great Lakes, and in 1988, she created a campaign to raise awareness and funding for children with disabilities through an organization known as Variety Village (formerly known as Variety Club).

Her name had come up before, but this time, it struck me differently. There was something there, something I needed to look into. Later that week, I found myself going back to her 1988 crossing of Lake Ontario. I needed answers—a clue as to where we went wrong with our crossing.

Why hadn't my attempt worked?

What had we missed?

I pulled up a chart that listed all the distances and times from Vicki's Great Lake crossings, and as I read through the numbers, the answer hit me like a truck: *distances!*

We had tried to cross Lake Ontario with a route that was 170 kilometres long. Vicki had crossed the lake using a 44.2-kilometre route. That meant we had taken on a course four times the length of Vicki's crossing.

As I looked at her numbers again—Lake Ontario, forty-four kilometres; Lake Erie, twenty-six kilometres; Lake Huron, seventy-five kilometres; Lake Superior, thirty-two kilometres; Lake Michigan, seventy-two kilometres. How had I missed it?!

Famous Swimmers on Lake Ontario

Marilyn Bell: Bell became the first person to swim across Lake Ontario in 1954 at just sixteen years old. Her successful swim from Youngstown, New York, to Toronto, Canada, took approximately twenty-one hours.[21]

Cindy Nicholas: Nicholas holds the record for the fastest female crossing of Lake Ontario, accomplished in 1974 with a time of 15 hours and 10 minutes. She later went on to swim across the English Channel numerous times, including the first double crossing of the Channel by a woman, earning her the nickname "Queen of the Channel."[22]

Vicki Keith: An accomplished marathon swimmer, Keith crossed Lake Ontario multiple times. In 1987, she became the first person to complete a double crossing of Lake Ontario.[23]

---

[21] Wikipedia Contributors. 2024. "Marilyn Bell." Wikipedia. Wikimedia Foundation. September 13, 2024. https://en.wikipedia.org/wiki/Marilyn_Bell.
[22] Wikipedia Contributors. 2024. "Cindy Nicholas." Wikipedia. Wikimedia Foundation. October 11, 2024. https://en.wikipedia.org/wiki/Cindy_Nicholas.
[23] Wikipedia Contributors. 2024. "Vicki Keith." Wikipedia. Wikimedia Foundation. August 7, 2024. https://en.wikipedia.org/wiki/Vicki_Keith.

I couldn't believe I hadn't seen it sooner.

My ego took a beating over the revelation that we'd essentially planned a crossing in the most difficult way possible.

That week, I walked down to Lake Ontario and sat along the shoreline, watching as the waves came in. It was a clear day, and I could literally see across the lake from Ontario to New York State.

That's when I knew I wasn't done with Lake Ontario. I had a new plan: to retry Lake Ontario using Vicki's 1988 route. But it wouldn't be just a one-crossing event. I would build a three-month campaign using all of her routes.

The longest of her crossings was seventy-five kilometres and we'd already covered that during my missed attempt, meaning that I already knew I was strong enough to last at least that long. I just needed to be mentally and physically strong enough to endure that *five* times.

This time, I was going to cross all five of the Great Lakes. Just like she had. One lake at a time.

* * *

I called Captain Keith to ask if I could bounce an idea off him. A few days later, I found myself sitting at his kitchen table, eating sushi with him, Sarah, and their son.

"I'm going to redo the Lake Ontario attempt," I said, trying not to let my chopsticks shake from how anxious I was.

The dinner table was quiet. They could tell there was more.

I continued, "But this time, I'm going to do all five Great Lakes . . . And I need your help."

He didn't say no. He didn't say anything. He just listened.

I blurted out everything I knew about Vicky's routes, where we had gone wrong, and why I already knew I could do this.

When I finished, I shoved a chicken teriyaki roll into my mouth and braced for rejection.

Anyone else might have told me I was crazy and tried to talk me out of it. But Keith was different. He was a big-picture guy. And he had always believed in me, whether I deserved it or not.

That day was no different. Keith and Sarah met me without question and gave me the same support and love they'd given me the first day we'd met.

By the time the plates were cleared from the table, I had pulled out the chart showing Vicki's crossings, and Keith had grabbed a map of Lake Ontario. We spread them all out across the dining room table and proceeded to go over what we had done previously and what we could do differently this time.

"I need your help," I told him honestly. I didn't want to do the campaign without him.

"Well, you have me for two crossings," Keith said. "I can't get out of work for all five, but you've got me for Lake Erie and Lake Ontario. And I'll help with the planning to make sure we do this right this time."

I wished I could have him for the whole campaign, but two of five was enough to make me feel like this was possible.

A wave of relief washed over me.

We immediately agreed that "rain or shine" firm dates were a bad idea. Instead, we would have a weather window—a week in which we would wait for the best day to make the attempt. Being flexible with the elements that were out of our control meant having more focus on the elements we could control—food, physical and mental health, navigation, strength building, and perseverance to complete the crossing.

With better weather, I could spend more time making forward momentum and less time fighting waves and currents.

At least, that was the theory.

* * *

The air grew cold, and the days shorter once again, but I barely noticed. I was laser-focused on the crossings and felt the momentum building inside me.

This time, I was going to focus on building the best possible team. I was grateful to have Keith, but I needed more. I brought on a nutritionist, a dietitian, and a personal trainer—Jonathan, Tanya, and Katia—all of whom volunteered their time to help me. My goal was simple but ambitious: I wanted to gain twenty pounds of muscle in the next six months.

Every morning, my alarm went off at 5:15 a.m., and by 5:30,

I was out of the house. I wanted to be the first person at the gym when it opened at 6:00. I lifted weights for an hour each day, pushing my body to its limits, and by 7:15, I was done.

A couple of years beforehand, I could barely walk from the living room to the bathroom on my own. But now, here I was—training for something bigger than myself, something that would make a real difference in the world.

Each step, each lift, and each hour in the gym reminded me of how far I'd come.

By Christmas, I was telling my family about the new campaign. I wasn't sure how surprised they'd be—after all, they knew I was training every day, and my mother had noticed the shifts in my attitude and routine. Still, I expected some pushback or at least hesitation.

Again, I was met with support. If they were nervous about me taking on this challenge, they didn't show it.

We talked about logistics, goals, and what we would do differently this time. I occasionally caught glimpses of concern in their eyes, but they were quickly replaced with excitement. They knew this wasn't just about crossing lakes—it was about proving something to myself. I wouldn't let them—or myself—down.

In January, I took my physical training up another notch by incorporating paddleboarding into my routine. The gym was great for building muscle, but nothing would prepare me for the lakes quite like being out on the water. Twice a week, I ventured out onto Lake Ontario, even when the temperatures dropped to -20°C. I'd borrowed a dry suit from my friend Sebastien and headed out into the icy water, looking more like an astronaut than a paddleboarder.

Many times, I was the only person out there. The lake was eerily quiet, with no boats, no people, just the sound of my paddle cutting through the water and the soft splash of the waves. I found myself enjoying the solitude. I was no longer afraid to be alone with my own thoughts. Instead, I looked forward to it.

As my physical and mental strength grew, so did my team. When I wasn't training, I was reaching out to potential boat captains, support crews, and even meteorologists who had covered the Lake Ontario crossing the previous year. Each conversation added another piece to the puzzle until, finally, I had a full team of people who believed in me and who were as invested in this campaign as I was.

I think of that winter in 2022 as a season of growth. Every day was spent building the foundations of the Great Lakes campaign—strengthening my body, refining my plans, and solidifying my support network. I spent countless hours finding sponsors and ticking things off the to-do list.

I discovered the power of admitting I needed help and asking for it. Instead of feeling embarrassed by my own perceived limitations, I was overwhelmed to see how many people jumped in without question, going out of their way to contribute to this massive goal of creating change.

There was a sense of urgency in everything I did, but also a quiet confidence growing inside me.

I reviewed what worked best during the first crossing in terms of finding outside support. I quickly realized that it was politicians.

So, I started contacting mayors' offices from across the province of Ontario requesting a meeting with myself and the founder of Jack.org, Eric Windeler.

Eric attended countless meetings with mayors in major cities during which I laid out the campaign routes and goals, and asked for their support.

On April 14, Eric met me in front of the LED Toronto sign in front of the fountain at Nathan Philip Square for a meeting at Toronto City Hall. With his bike in tow and his biker apparel, he looked like he was about to cycle across Canada. I was anxious about the meeting—it was the biggest one I'd had to date.

When we were called into the office of Mayor John Tory, I was wearing my Jack.org T-shirt that read, "This is what a mental health advocate looks like."

The mayor opened our conversation by eloquently discussing the impacts of mental health since the COVID-19 pandemic and how it was affecting the people of Toronto and youth in Canada.

I was impressed by how knowledgeable and passionate the mayor was. It wasn't long before he offered his support, pledging to do whatever he could to help the campaign.

Later that day, his team posted a photo across his social media accounts with Eric and me standing in front of the flags in his office, announcing that in two months time, I would attempt to become the first person to paddleboard across the Great Lakes to raise awareness for Jack.org and youth mental health with a note that Toronto was cheering for me.

This time, we didn't have to announce the upcoming campaign. The Toronto mayor had done it for us.

I prepared to go into PR mode, bracing for the feedback and interview requests, but instead, I was met with silence. The mayor of the largest city in Canada had told the world about our campaign and no one seemed to be listening.

Maybe no one believed I could do it because of my failure the first time.

* * *

By April, everything was in place for the campaign.

Captain Keith remained my go-to for the crossings of Lake Erie and Lake Ontario, and we lined up charter boats for Lake Huron and Lake Superior. We were still working on a charter boat for the Lake Michigan crossing, but we were farther ahead than we'd been a year before.

We brought in two cinematographers, Matt and Joe, who had personal ties to mental health and wanted to help. With long hair and laid-back attitudes, they both had the surfer look.

They both understood the gravity of what we were trying to accomplish, and their previous experience filming on the Great Lakes would be invaluable. Matt, in particular, had already shot short films of surfers on the lakes and knew how quickly the weather could change. His experience with navigation and weather patterns would come in very handy.

Keith and I spent part of nearly every day on the water together, fine-tuning my technique and timing me for speed.

By May, I was paddling at an average of 3.5 to 4 kilometres per hour. In my first Lake Ontario crossing attempt, I'd struggled to maintain two kilometres per hour.

The time spent training with Keith was an escape from the intensity of campaign planning. It reminded me of how much I loved being out on the water, why I loved paddleboarding, and why I had started this in the first place—because out on the water, I felt *alive*.

Around that same time, I got a call from Liz Braun at the *Toronto Sun*, apologizing for not covering the Lake Ontario attempt the year before. I had no idea who she was at first, but by the end of the conversation, I felt like I had made a new friend. Liz was enthusiastic about the Great Lakes campaign and promised to cover the story this time around.

That same week, I was invited to Variety Village, the non-profit organization that Vicki Keith had worked with, to meet with their president, Archie Allison. I was also going to meet Vicki Keith herself.

I toured the facility, meeting the Variety Club team and learning more about their work. And then, there she was—Vicki Keith, the woman who had inspired this entire campaign. She was warm and kind, with the energy of someone who still lived and breathed the water. She was fit, and it was clear she still swam regularly.

We sat down in a boardroom, and I finally had the chance to talk to her about my plans. We discussed the logistics of the Great Lakes campaign in detail—routes, distances, support crews, weather windows, and nutrition. She was excited, and her excitement fuelled my own. I could see the spark in her eyes when she talked about the lakes, especially Lake Superior.

I wondered if I'd feel the same way, if there would be one lake that stood out for me, or if they'd all blend into one great challenge.

As we wrapped up the meeting, she gave me the most important advice of all: rely on your team. Lean on them. Let them support you in the way they are meant to. This is a lesson that would inevitably save me countless times in my life. I just didn't know it yet.

Soon, I met with over twenty different Ontario mayors to ask for their support.

Media finally started to pick up the story again, and I embraced it. I was grateful for the coverage, bringing attention to the organization and to the cause.

The morning shows in Toronto were the first to request

interviews. That meant being in the studio or out on the water with their film crews early in the mornings.

PR didn't drain me as much as the first crossing, but it took its toll, and I knew I had to protect my health. My recovery from Ramsay Hunt syndrome was still a work in progress, so I focused on balance above all else.

Being with Keith in the evenings out on the water was a nice break from the spotlight, giving me time to train and focus on what was really important.

I was ready to show the world that the failed Lake Ontario attempt wasn't the end of my story.

It was only the beginning.

A LESSON IN SAGACITY

Crossing "rain or shine" was a decision based more on keeping to a date on the calendar than on critical elements, information, or experience.

Failing that first Lake Ontario crossing was a wake-up call that we had a lot to learn about what we still had to learn, that we needed to bring on people who had the experience and wisdom we didn't, and that we needed to accept what we could and could not control.

When I speak about leadership and teamwork to corporations and organizations, we often discuss "sagacity." Sagacity is a powerful yet often overlooked trait that means to have (and seek) foresight, discernment, and keen perception. Having sagacity means making thoughtful decisions based on information, experience, and wise predictions rather than impulse. You're better able to adapt to change—often without introducing higher risk. This capacity to see beyond the immediate challenges is what distinguishes truly effective leaders and individuals, and it is a trait that I strive to exude every day.

The wisdom that comes from sagacity makes complex problems a lot easier to solve. You have built a deeper understanding of the issue at hand and can more easily see potential consequences.

After Lake Ontario, we knew we needed to build a team with sagacity.

CHAPTER 7

LAKE ERIE | TEAM SUPPORT

On the morning of May 26, Keith and I packed up and left Whitby, Ontario, bound for Crystal Beach, a small community perched along Lake Erie, 207 kilometres to the southwest. There was an underlying sense of anticipation in the air. We had five to seven days before attempting the first crossing of the Great Lakes, and with that came the weight of preparation. Crystal Beach would be our base camp, and we knew that everything had to be ready.

This was also the first time I had driven since the Ramsay Hunt syndrome diagnosis. I can't describe the feeling of complete freedom that came with being able to drive again.

Just one week beforehand, we didn't even know how we would get from point A to point B on land, how we would pick up supplies, refill the boats, get team members to hotels, move from one shore to another . . . until Mazda Canada saved the day.

I had just spent months reaching out to a multitude of Canadian Car Manufacturers and dealerships from across the province in hopes of sponsorship. Many said no. Others didn't bother to reply at all. I'd just about given up when Mazda Canada offered to donate a brand new 2023 Mazda CX 50 sports utility vehicle for the campaign.

Having Mazda believe in me and this campaign enough to attach their brand to it and to mental health gave us all the confidence boost we needed when we needed it most.

The vehicle had a roof rack that could hold my twenty-one-foot board, a deep trunk for storage and all the bags and equipment of my team.

The Mazda team wrapped the vehicle in *"Driven for Change"* and Jack.org marketing. It was perfect.

Keith and I made three stops along that first drive, each one a reminder of the kindness and support we'd received from people who believed in what we were doing. At our first stop, we picked up crates of fresh fruit and vegetables, all donated by local grocers.

The next stop was Cobb's Bread, where they handed over boxes of freshly baked goods.

Our final stop was at a deli in St. Catharines, where we collected an assortment of meats to feed the team during the Lake Erie crossing.

By the time we reached the house in Crystal Beach, the Mazda was filled to the brim with food and supplies. The house had been generously donated by Re/Max Canada Realtors through a connection from my friend Jennifer, who was also a paddleboarder. It was the perfect base of operations for the team. It wasn't beachfront, but it had that unmistakable beachhouse feel—white walls, blue accents, starfish, and sand dollar decor accents.

When Matt, our cinematographer from Michigan, arrived and met Keith for the first time, they hit it off right away. The three of us spent the evening setting up, hauling in supplies, and making plans for the week ahead.

Keith, Matt, and I piled into the Mazda and drove about twenty minutes to Niagara Falls to meet some of my friends who had travelled up to watch the crossing.

Seven of us went to a steakhouse that evening to celebrate my birthday. We swapped stories and laughs. Matt's passage through the US-Canada border had been its own saga, with Canadian customs curious about his equipment and why he was travelling with so many cameras and drones.

We talked about the days ahead and mapped out the plan for tomorrow. It was hard to believe that we were finally here, standing on the cusp of crossing the first Great Lake from Point Sturgeon, New York, to Crystal Beach, Ontario.

Afterward, we made a trip down to the falls to watch fireworks illuminate the night sky.

As the sky lit up with bursts of light and colour, I tried to embrace the moment. I was feeling the weight of the crossing, but having friends and team members around me who I trusted took the edge off of it.

The fireworks started to taper down, and we agreed to call it a night in exchange for a good night's sleep. My friends headed home with promises to see me on shore the following day. The team and I went back to our Crystal Beach home base.

In bed, I checked my phone one last time. Matt and Keith had already assured me the weather was optimal, but it was nice to also get a message from Ross Hull, the meteorologist at Global News, saying the same.

In so many ways, I knew this crossing was nothing like the Lake Ontario crossing. This time I had a team who knew their roles and were as invested in our goal as I was. Also, I'd planned this better.

Better yet, I was stronger, physically and mentally. That would help me sustain myself out there if the weather decided to turn and the water got rough.

It was close to midnight when I closed my eyes.

When my alarm went off at six o'clock the next morning, I wasn't tired. It was still dark outside, but I felt energized and excited.

It's crossing day.

Members of my team began arriving. I greeted them on the street before going over the plan together in person for the first time.

> LAKE ERIE is known to be large, shallow, and temperamental. With a max depth of 64 metres, storms could form fast. It has a surface area of 25,667 square kilometres, making it the fourth-largest Great Lake. Erie's north shore hugs Ontario in Canada, and its southern side runs along Ohio, Pennsylvania, and New York in the US.[24]

Keith, Matt, and I got in the Mazda, pointed it to the beach, and led the procession of our three cars filled with our team toward the marina.

Jennifer stepped out of one of the cars and greeted me with a hug. "Are you ready?" she asked, studying my face for signs that we should call it off.

"Ready!" I beamed.

My trainers, Tanya and Katia, arrived with Oliver.

There were eight people in total on the support boat.

The idea was to have more support than needed. We planned to gauge what was needed from this crossing—"the learning crossing"—for the ones still ahead.

The support boat left the Canadian side and travelled to Point Sturgeon, New York, with the paddleboard attached to the side, ripping through the water.

The mood among the team was light. Laughter filled the air,

---

[24] Wikipedia Contributors. 2024. "Lake Erie." Wikipedia. Wikimedia Foundation. September 19, 2024. https://en.wikipedia.org/wiki/Lake_Erie.

and despite the early hour, there was an energy that couldn't be ignored. We were ready.

At 8:30 a.m., we neared the New York shore, the boat engines slowed, and the paddleboard was lowered into the water. I climbed onto it and took a moment to ground myself before launching.

The water was still, and as I began paddling, I could hear my team cheering "Woo hoo" and "Goooo Miiiike" and "You've got this" from the boat.

I raised my paddle in the air to show I was ready.

My mantra echoed in my head: *This is not Lake Ontario.*

Lake Ontario was a lesson I needed to learn. It had taught me all the information I needed to get me where I was now.

Vicki had once been in this same spot thirty-four years before. I thought about how nervous and excited she must have been.

The first few hours were smooth. My body and mind were feeling good, and I trailed the boat closely, positioning myself on the left side so that I could hear them better through my good ear (most of my hearing loss from RHS was in my right).

I was close enough to the support boat that I could hear the music on the boat—a mixture of top-40 hits, pop, and country music. The music and my team's energy were motivating.

Every thirty minutes, a bell rang, signalling that it was time to paddle over for hydration—my pack was refilled with a mix of water and Gatorade. I'd grab a quick bite, usually a sandwich or fruit, and then head back out. The sun beat down with all its might, and by noon, I was sweating heavily inside the black wet suit.

By early afternoon, the rip currents became very strong and took the support boat and myself off course, pushing us east.

My first instinct was to panic.

This is not Lake Ontario.

Fear of failure is a powerful force, one that affects us mentally and physically.

What if I can't do this?

"Focus on following the boat, Mike," someone said from the deck of the boat.

I did as I was told while the team navigated us through the currents as best as possible. We weren't going in a straight line anymore, but we were making some progress.

For the next two hours, the currents pushed us, and we pushed back harder.

I focused on moving my paddle through the water on one side, then the other, back and forth.

The shoreline was in sight, a strip of land in the distance. Because the lake is deceiving, the land looked much closer than it was, so no matter how hard I paddled, it felt like we were stuck in place, moving sideways instead of forward. It started to mess with my head, making each stroke more of an effort.

By late afternoon, after what felt like an eternity, I started to see silhouettes on the Ontario beach ahead. I blinked a few times to be sure I wasn't seeing things.

Soon, I could hear them too—muffled voices in the distance. We were almost there.

The last bell rang, and I was pulled in for a final pep talk. Even though we were close to the finish line, the sun, heat, and exertion had my team worrying about hydration.

"How many times have you gone to the bathroom in the last half hour?" someone asked.

I admitted to averaging two or three times every half hour. And given the circumstances and to save time, I just let it run down my legs as I paddled.

They filled my hydration pack with Gatorade one last time and passed it back to me. I put it over my sunburned shoulders, which were red as a firetruck, and was given one final pep talk by the team.

"This is it. This is the moment you've been training for. This is one in five, and you're about to do it. Go get it!"

With a racing heart, I pushed through the final stretch. Thirty minutes felt like an hour. I was so excited to get off the board and onto the shore; it was excruciating to maintain patience.

The beach voices grew louder. I could feel the excitement of my team.

I pulled up my wet suit to cover my chest and arms.

Keith stepped out from the helm and said, "The team is

going to head to the marina on the tender. It's time for you to paddle ahead. They'll meet you on shore.

The water grew shallower, and when I was about twenty feet from shore, I jumped off the board and ran through the water, pulling it behind me. My legs burned, but the adrenaline coursing through my veins carried me forward.

Some people in the crowd had waded into the water to meet me, but I knew the sand was the true finish line.

I could make out the face of my dad and aimed directly for him. He has his phone out, recording the second my feet stepped onto Canadian land. It was 4:30 p.m. in Crystal Beach, Ontario.

Dad hugged me hard. Friends, supporters, team members, and government officials were cheering and clapping. I was dizzy and could barely discern one person from another, but that didn't matter. I felt the love surrounding me.

We did it. We crossed the first of the Great Lakes.

The wave of emotion hit me so hard it took my breath away.

I was presented with a certificate by Mayor Wayne Redekop as he officially welcomed me to Crystal Beach.

We spoke briefly about the mental health crisis in Ontario. His words resonated with me. This wasn't just about crossing lakes—it was about shining a light on something bigger.

That night, after dinner, I sat with Keith and Matt on the porch of our gifted beach house. We reflected on the day, the highs and lows, about the team's incredible support and how far we'd come since the Lake Ontario attempt. The stars shone above us, and for the first time in a long while, I allowed myself to feel proud.

When I crawled into bed that night, the heat radiated off my back and shoulders. I was alone and smiling bigger than I had in a very long time, knowing that I had just done something really special.

Our team did something really special.

A LESSON IN TEAM BUILDING

There's a saying, "If you want to go fast, go alone. If you want to go far, go together." And I had a long way to go to cross all five Great Lakes safely.

Going back to the water and trying again meant learning from previous mistakes and doing things differently this time. This time:

- I wasn't afraid to ask for help.
- I reached out to people who had experience, vision, and sagacity and who wouldn't be afraid to collaborate on anything and everything with the rest of the team.
- I purposely "overstaffed" while we tested out how many people we truly needed.

- I embraced people who came into it with a clear belief in the vision I had for this campaign.
- I welcomed team members who were supportive, accountable, eager to help others, and a positive contribution to the morale and motivation of all of us.

The lessons learned and implemented from the first attempt created a completely different experience.

CHAPTER 8

LAKE HURON | LESSONS IN LIGHT

As we arrived home from the Lake Erie crossing, the headlines began to spread.

"Paddleboarder Crosses Lake Erie in World-First Achievement," they read. Every news outlet seemed to be covering it. When I turned on *Breakfast Television*, Sid Seixeiro and Dina Pugliese were talking about the crossing during their segment, "The Bright Spot." They rang a bell, and the studio cheered in celebration.

Despite all the attention, I needed to rest. I had promised myself and the team that I would. So, I turned off my phone, shut down my emails, and spent the day doing as little as possible. At least, that was the plan. The problem with downtime is that it gives your mind room to wander, and mine was already moving ahead to Lake Huron.

There was still so much to do. Part of me felt guilty. How could I rest when there was another lake waiting to be crossed? How could I rest knowing there was still so much work ahead?

When I finally turned my phone back on, the outpouring of support was overwhelming. Messages flooded in from all over, social media posts from people I didn't even know, cheering me on. Municipalities across Ontario had shared messages of congratulations. Their mayors and city councillors posted about the crossing. I responded to some, thanked as many as I could, but soon enough, I had to put the phone down again.

There was no time to bask in the afterglow. In just a few days, we'd be heading for Lake Huron. It was the second largest of the Great Lakes, and for us, it was also the longest crossing in our campaign.

> LAKE HURON is the second largest of the Great Lakes by surface area, covering approximately 59,600 square kilometres. The lake has an average depth of 59 metres and a maximum depth of 229 metres. It has the longest shoreline of all the Great Lakes, including its 30,000 islands. The largest island in any freshwater lake in the world, Manitoulin Island, is located in Lake Huron.[25]

Having just finished the shortest crossing, Lake Huron felt like going from a warm-up to jumping into the deep end.

The plan was to head to Harbor Beach, Michigan, by

---

25   Wikipedia Contributors. 2024. "Lake Huron." Wikipedia. Wikimedia Foundation. August 23, 2024. https://en.wikipedia.org/wiki/Lake_Huron.

June 7, just nine days after the Erie crossing, and position ourselves for the next leg. This would be a significant leap, and I knew it.

Crossing the border into Michigan came with its own stress. The immigration officer was full of questions about the paddleboard strapped to the roof of the Mazda and why a team of people was heading across the border. Each inquiry made me more anxious, irrationally fearing they'd turn us away for some small, unpredictable reason. But in the end, we passed through without much trouble, and a few hours later, we pulled into a small motel. The place felt like a relic from another time, outdated and weathered—kind of like the Bates Motel from *Psycho*. But Carl, the man who ran the place, was friendly and welcoming.

That night, we grabbed pizza and wings from the local shop Carl recommended and ate outside at the picnic tables in front of our rooms. The team—Matt, Joe, and the others—was glued to their phones, checking weather patterns and making sure we had a window to cross in the coming days. There was a calm among us, a quiet confidence. We had one crossing under our belts, and it felt like we were in a good place. But there was one thing missing—Captain Keith.

Keith had been a central part of the Lake Erie crossing, and his absence was noticeable. With his work commitments keeping him away, we had chartered a boat captain to take his place, but it wasn't the same. I missed Keith's steady presence, his humour, and the way he kept things light even in moments of tension.

He'd love this, I thought, *sitting outside, laughing, and sharing stories with the team.*

But he wasn't here, and that made the whole thing feel incomplete.

The next morning, we were at breakfast when the logistics coordinator's phone rang, and he stepped outside to take the call. I could tell from the look on his face when he came back that something was wrong. The boat and drivers we had chartered to cross Lake Huron had suffered a catastrophic engine failure near Detroit. They wouldn't be able to make it. Just like that, we were without a boat and a captain for the longest, most critical crossing of the campaign.

Without a boat, we would be grounded.

We called Eric from Jack.org, updated him on the situation, and ran through possible solutions, but none of them seemed viable. In a moment of frustration, I even suggested making the crossing without a support boat, just me and my board. That idea was shot down quickly, and rightfully so. We needed a boat. Without one, the entire plan was at risk of falling apart.

We shifted into crisis mode, pulling out our phones and laptops, trying to find a solution. Two members of the team drove to the local marina to search for a boat while the rest of us began calling marinas across Michigan, Ohio, and even

Indiana. But the response was the same every time: "We're fully booked. We don't have anything available."

It felt a lot like the months before Lake Ontario, when I sent out hundreds of emails and calls, only to be met with rejection after rejection.

By the next morning, we were at breakfast once again, and I realized something: we were too focused on the fact that we were departing from the US side.

"Why not call marinas on the Canadian side?" I asked the team at the table. "After all, we will be landing in Canada, so it makes sense to have a boat and captain from Ontario. Plus, they wouldn't have to make the long trip back after the crossing; they'd already be home."

I didn't know it then, but that thought would change everything.

We started calling marinas in towns along Lake Huron's eastern shore: Kincardine, Goderich, and others. Hours passed, and then, out of nowhere, we got a callback. The man on the other end introduced himself as Jim Peever. He ran the Maitland Valley Marina in Goderich, Ontario, and after hearing about our situation, he said he'd be willing to help.

He hadn't even put his boat in the water yet for the season, but he was willing to check with Canadian Border Services and the American Coast Guard to see if he could make it happen.

An hour later, the phone rang again. Jim was on the line,

and he had news: "I've got the all-clear from both sides. When do you need me?"

We couldn't believe it. We had a boat. We had a captain. The entire team erupted in celebration, jumping up and down with joy. That evening, Jim left the town of Goderich in his motorboat, *The Why Knot*, and crossed Lake Huron on his own, arriving at Harbor Beach, Michigan, just after sunset.

While I slept, my team met Jim and loaded the boat with everything we'd need—equipment, food, fuel. Captain Jim had saved us, and I hadn't even met him yet.

At 4:30 a.m. the next morning, my alarm went off. I checked my phone and saw a message from my dad: "Let me know what time you're leaving."

I texted back, "I'll launch at 6 a.m."

"Good luck and Godspeed," he replied. I could hear his warm voice as I read the words. I smiled and got up to prepare for one of the biggest days of my life.

By 5:30 a.m., we were at the marina, and I met Jim Peever for the first time. He poked his head out of the boat, and the first thing I noticed was his big, bushy beard. Because of this, he reminded me of Keith. I thanked him over and over for stepping in to save the crossing. He humbly waved it off like it was nothing before launching into the rules of his boat and reminding us of the dangers ahead. He was a no-nonsense man, but there was a warmth in his demeanour that put me at ease.

I spent a few moments alone at the Harbor Beach shoreline,

standing beside a historical marker dedicated to Vicki Keith's epic swim across Lake Huron in 1988. It was erected in 1990 by the citizens of Harbor Beach in Huron County, Michigan and read:

> *At 7 A.M. Sunday, July 17, 1988, 27 year old Vicki Keith departed from Harbor Beach on an epic swim across Lake Huron. Vicki swam on through July 17, July 18, and onward into the early hours of Tuesday, July 19th. She arrived on the sand beach adjacent to the harbour at the port of Goderich, Ontario to a cheering crowd of 400 at 5:55 a.m. after swimming for almost two days, Vicki completed the swim by using her trademark butterfly stroke for the last half mile from the outer break wall to the beach. After being blown off course for a time Vicki swam a total of 48 miles over a period of 46 hours and 55 minutes.*

As I stood there, reading the words, I couldn't help but feel a connection to her, a sense of shared purpose. We were both pushing ourselves to the limit, testing our endurance against the vastness of these waters.

At 7 a.m. the drone flew overhead, signalling that the team was ready. I stepped into the water, climbed onto my board, and began paddling out. *Here we go again* I thought, as the vast expanse of Lake Huron stretched out before me. But I knew this was going to be nothing like before.

Like Lake Erie, the first few hours were smooth. Jim set a steady pace, and I kept to the right side of the boat, falling into a rhythm. If we maintained three kilometres per hour, we'd be across in twenty-five hours. But by 10 a.m., the skies began to darken. The blue horizon turned a deep grey, the winds picked up, and the water grew choppy. For the next three hours, I fought the currents and waves.

I paddled furiously to keep pace with the boat. It was exhausting. Every muscle in my body screamed for relief, but the only option was to push forward.

The bell rang every thirty minutes, calling me to the boat for hydration and a shake. Each hand off was risky because of the waves. It would have been so easy to get thrown into the boat. But we managed.

Still, as the hours wore on, I could feel my energy draining.

At 2 p.m. the wind changed again, this time pushing us backward. The boat tried to shield me, but even with its protection, the relentless gusts made it nearly impossible for me to stand.

I switched to a seated position and paddled that way, knowing it would be slightly slower but continuing to do my best to stay on course.

My mind wandered to the ships I could see in the distance, their silhouettes cutting through the horizon. Lake Huron was no joke—it has a rich history of shipwrecks, with the Thunder Bay National Marine Sanctuary protecting many of these underwater sites, offering opportunities for diving and exploration.

It was 6 p.m. before the wind finally began to die down, and the blue sky returned. The team and I shared stories, trying to lift my spirits. We played silly games like assigning barnyard animals to each team member based on their personality traits.

I got to choose Captain Jim's animal, and he became a sheepdog—steady, protective, and always on guard. Sheepdogs are intelligent, agile, and invaluable. The sheepdog has three main responsibilities: herding the sheep from one place to another, guarding the flock from predators, and managing the flock during frightening activities, helping to keep them calm and organized.

Once night fell, the temperature dropped rapidly.

I knew from research that Lake Huron had the longest shoreline of all the Great Lakes, not to mention the host of thirty-thousand islands. But by then, all I could see was darkness.

The team fitted me with lights, attaching them to my hat, arms, and legs so they could see me. Then, they pointed a powerful production light at the water, illuminating the path ahead so that I could see my way. The light drew me toward it like a beacon.

The cold set in quickly. The damp air soaked through my clothes, and soon, I was shivering uncontrollably. I didn't say anything to the team at first, for fear they would call off the crossing, but by midnight, I couldn't hide it anymore. They could see my shaking from the deck.

Joe, who had taken the night shift at the back of the boat, called me over and handed me new gloves, a hat, and a winter coat.

Joe and I talked through the night, our conversation ranging from movies to books to his family and little girl. We talked about our shared appreciation for *The Dark Knight* and all things in the *Batman* universe. It was a distraction, something to keep my mind off the biting cold and the endless hours ahead.

We talked for hours until I broke down and admitted to him that I couldn't feel my fingers.

I trusted Joe, and he saw me through most of the night while the other team members slept and took breaks down below in the cabin.

I was so tired at that point; my eyes were having trouble discerning what I was seeing as we crossed through the busy shipping lanes.

"What are those lights ahead?" I asked Joe.

He followed my gaze. "That's a lighthouse," he explained. But that didn't make any sense because I was seeing multiple lighthouses, and they were spinning like a carousel.

I was hallucinating.

* * *

When the sun came up, the world looked right again. I'd made it through the hardest part of this. We all had.

Seeing the shoreline gave me new energy.

Calls were made to my family to let them know we had made it through the night and would be arriving on the shores of Goderich in about six hours.

My team read messages from social media to keep my spirits lifted and keep me going.

At 10 a.m., Captain Jim called the Canadian Coast Guard on the radio to alert them that we were approaching the Canadian side. They sent out an escort to help guide us in.

The sight of the red and white coast guard boat was very exciting. (By then, I could also see the lighthouse and realized there was no carousel.)

At 11:30 a.m., after over twenty-eight hours on the water, I arrived at the beach in Goderich. Unlike the triumphant sprint onto Crystal Beach just two weeks earlier, this landing was different. My feet were pruned, waterlogged to the point that I couldn't put pressure on them. Walking was agony, but I was just so relieved to have completed the crossing that I kept going, using my paddle as a cane to help me hobble out of the water.

My dad was the first to reach me, grabbing me in a tight hug. I fell into his arms and hung onto him for support.

A small crowd had gathered—family, friends, reporters, and Mayor John Grace of Goderich. I smiled for as many photos as I could before the ambulance arrived. It had been called from the boat to check on my foot. They checked me out and told me to stay off my foot for a few days but that I would be okay. They also checked my hydration and said, "Whatever you're doing for hydration, keep doing that!"

A LESSON IN LIGHTKEEPING

Lake Huron ended up hitting close to home due to all the ways it tried to pull me back to the night that depression nearly took my life. During Huron, it was a long, tiring, dark crossing. I was spiralling. My mind began playing tricks on me, like imagining I was surrounded by people who were there for me yet fighting a feeling of loneliness and isolation.

Why did I feel that way?

As I look back now, I realize that it was the darkness that triggered my depression. Stress hormones such as cortisol often peak at night, pulling you down and affecting not just your mental health but your physical health as well. Add in exhaustion and a lack of sleep, and all of a sudden, I was on the brink of breaking.

What kept me from drowning?

I had my team. My Lightkeepers. Joe kept me talking, team members shared stories, they each shone their lights for me, and by the end of the night, they had each become the beacon I so desperately needed to lead me through the darkness. I would not have made it without them.

If one in five people experience mental illness in any given year, imagine how game-changing it would be to empower the other four in that statistic to act as beacons—Lightkeepers—for the ones who are lost. It would change the way we look at that statistic.

Every person in the midst of a struggle to keep their head above water deserves what I had on that night in the middle of Lake Huron—a team of Lightkeepers to hold space for them, provide safe harbour, guide them, and act as beacons to pull them through the most difficult times.

CHAPTER 9

LAKE SUPERIOR | SOLUTION-SEEKING

The days following our return from Lake Huron were slow, almost painfully so. My body ached in places I hadn't known could hurt. The exhaustion that had been creeping in during the crossing finally caught up with me.

The paramedics had told me to stay off my feet for a few days, and for once, I listened. I didn't have much choice; the swelling in my right foot had worsened, and my entire body was screaming for rest.

Even though my mind raced, I couldn't ignore the physical toll the crossing had taken. Muscles were tight, my joints stiff, and the mental fatigue from fighting Lake Huron was harder to shake than I'd anticipated.

Every time I closed my eyes, I was back in the dark waters, feeling the strain in my arms, core, and legs as I paddled through the cold, unrelenting wind.

But just as I settled into some semblance of recovery, the news broke. Justin Bieber, the world-famous Canadian singer, had announced that he too was suffering from Ramsay Hunt syndrome. Suddenly, people began to understand what I'd been dealing with. For months, my condition felt invisible to the world—something only I and a handful of others truly understood. But with Bieber's diagnosis, Ramsay Hunt syndrome was front and centre in the news. And with that came the media attention.

Requests for interviews came pouring in. Journalists who hadn't cared much before suddenly wanted to hear about my own experience, about how I had managed to push myself across these massive bodies of water while battling a condition that left me feeling weak and disoriented on my worst days.

Jack.org saw this as an opportunity to bring more attention to youth mental health, and I agreed. Still, the weight of it all was intense, and not every request was respectful.

Some media outlets wanted answers right away. Others were more respectful of boundaries, genuinely wanting to spread awareness and help those dealing with similar struggles. I tried to focus on the positive. This wasn't just about me—it was about helping kids and teens across Canada access the mental health services they needed. The spotlight wasn't comfortable, but it could do some good.

While I navigated the media whirlwind, the next crossing loomed ahead. The plan was clear: Lake Erie, Lake Huron, Lake Michigan, Lake Superior, and finally, Lake Ontario. But the next crossing—Lake Michigan—soon became a logistical nightmare.

For months, we had been trying to secure a charter boat that could act as my support vehicle for the crossing. But nothing was lining up.

The weather window was our first obstacle. It was going to fall right over the July 4 holiday weekend in the US, which meant that every available boat was booked solid. Fishermen and tourists filled the waters, and no one wanted to give up their prime holiday spots to help us cross Lake Michigan. With each passing day, the pressure mounted.

We had support boats lined up for both Lake Superior and Lake Ontario, but the Michigan leg of the campaign was starting to feel cursed.

We expanded our search. We looked in Illinois, Indiana, Ohio, and even as far as Missouri and Iowa. Still, no boats.

It was Matt, our logistics guy, who suggested we check the weather on Lake Superior instead. He and Keith had been going back and forth about whether it made sense to keep pushing for Michigan or, instead, to pivot.

The more we talked about it, the more we realized that, even if we did find a boat for Lake Michigan, the weather wasn't going to cooperate. The winds were high, the water was rough, and everything pointed to a miserable attempt.

Lake Superior was the calm option, despite its reputation for the opposite.

> LAKE SUPERIOR is the largest of the Great Lakes. It's the largest freshwater lake by surface area in the world, covering 82,100 square kilometres, with 4,387 kilometres of shoreline, which includes its many islands. It is famous for its fierce storms, including the one that sank the Edmund Fitzgerald, killing all twenty-nine crew members aboard.[26]

Over twenty-four hours, we changed all of our plans, abandoning Lake Michigan—for now, at least—to set our sights on Superior.

The team scrambled into action. A seventeen-hour drive across northern Ontario and Michigan into Wisconsin was hastily mapped out, accommodations were secured, and Captain Joe, who was scheduled to help us with the Lake Superior crossing, confirmed that he'd be ready earlier than expected.

The drive was gruelling, more so because we were all still worn down from the previous weeks. Long road trips had always been challenging for me, and though I did some of the driving, the familiar waves of vertigo that came with Ramsay Hunt syndrome hit me hard after a few hours.

We took turns behind the wheel. I tried to keep my mind off my nausea and focused on what was ahead. We ended up

---

[26] Jodie. 2022. "The Fateful Journey - Great Lakes Shipwreck Historical Society." Great Lakes Shipwreck Historical Society. October 14, 2022. https://shipwreckmuseum.com/the-fateful-journey/.

breaking the drive up into three days to accommodate my challenges.

Lake Superior—the one I'd been most afraid of, the one I'd heard so much about since childhood, full of tumultuous waves, shipwrecks including the SS Edmund Fitzgerald, and cold, unpredictable waters—was now our next challenge.

We arrived in Sudbury, Ontario, late in the evening. That night, the team was treated to dinner at MIC Eatery and Pub. MIC stood for Made in Canada, and the restaurant was decorated with patriotic gear and photos of Canadian icons.

The staff knew about my story, and they came over to talk to us at our table. They asked about the crossings and seemed to genuinely care about what we were doing. It was moments like those, when people showed genuine interest and support, which reminded me why I was doing this.

As we left, we stopped in the parking lot for photos with the owners and some of the serving team in front of the Mazda with the board tied to the roof.

The next morning, we were up early and headed to Cora's for breakfast. With July 1 (Canada Day) being the next day, the restaurant was filled with red and white balloons, and all the servers were wearing red cowboy hats.

Our server was very chatty.

"I could never do your job, having to be all smiles at the break of dawn!" I laughed, grateful for her cheerfulness.

Throughout our breakfast, she asked where we were from and where we were going. We fill her in about the crossings.

"I knew I recognized you! I saw your story on the news!" she said.

When it came time for her to clear our plates, we asked for the bill.

"It's been taken care of by one of our other guests," she said and winked at me.

The entire restaurant now knew. I found out who our sponsor was, went over to him, and shook his hand. We took a photo together, which, of course, started a series of photos with all of the servers and a few more guests. It was good to see that our campaign for awareness and change was being noticed by so many.

The drive that day was fun. We stopped to meet with some reporters to answer a mountain of questions and then proceeded to cross the border at Sault Ste. Marie into the US.

In Michigan, we stopped at the Great Lakes Shipwreck Museum. It was part distraction and part confrontation with the fear that had been lurking in the back of my mind.

The museum, located on the shores of Lake Superior at Whitefish Point, is dedicated to preserving the history of shipwrecks that had occurred in these treacherous waters. The exhibit on the "SS Edmund Fitzgerald," one of the most famous shipwrecks in Great Lakes history, struck a chord with me. The ship had gone down in a storm in 1975, killing all twenty-nine crew members on board. The bell from the ship had been recovered and was now the centrepiece of the museum's collection. Standing there, staring at that bell, I felt a mixture of awe and fear. Lake Superior was powerful, and while we weren't planning to cross in the middle of a storm, the unpredictability couldn't be ignored.

We were in the room dedicated to the SS Edmund Fitzgerald exhibit when we met a family from Minnesota. They sounded like they were straight out of the movie *Fargo*, and I smiled, recognizing the accent immediately.

They told us they were on a family vacation to Canada. When they found out where we were headed, they were shocked that we would attempt to cross Lake Superior. Their expressions, combined with being in front of the Edmund Fitzgerald exhibit, made me instantly anxious.

When we began talking about how this was all in support of youth mental health programs and services, the father tuned out of the conversation. It was a reminder that not everyone saw this as a need.

On the way out of the museum, we went through the gift shop. I spotted a small lapel pin that could be worn on a suit jacket. It was gold and shaped like a bell with the inscription, "The Edmund Fitzgerald." I bought it thinking that if I wore it, it would be a nice nod to history.

Maybe the Edmund Fitzgerald crew would keep me company and give me some luck out there.

> The SS Edmund Fitzgerald was a Great Lakes freighter built in 1958 by Great Lakes Engineering Works in River Rouge, Michigan. It is thought that the ship had come up on a storm with near-hurricane-force winds and waves up to 11 metres (35 feet). Captain McSorley's last message was said to be, "We are holding our own." It was transmitted at around 7:10 p.m. on November 10, 1975. No distress signal was ever sent. It is estimated to have sunk between 7:15 and 7:30 p.m. in Canadian waters, 163 metres below the surface of Lake Superior, broken in two.[27]

We spent that night in Christmas, Michigan, and, as you can imagine, the town was quite small and Christmas-themed. Santas and reindeer lined the highway leading into and through town. It could have been right out of a Hallmark movie. Our motel for the night was right beside a casino which, when we peeked inside, looked like Christmas threw up all over it.

We had some dinner and walked down to the lake to watch the sunset. It lit up the sky with oranges, pinks, and purples. The Lake Superior crossing was projected to take fifteen hours, so if all went according to plan, we wouldn't see the sunset during

---

27   Jodie. 2022. "The Fateful Journey - Great Lakes Shipwreck Historical Society." Great Lakes Shipwreck Historical Society. October 14, 2022. https://shipwreckmuseum.com/the-fateful-journey/.

the crossing to Minnesota. But we probably would see one while crossing back to Wisconsin in the boat.

I went off on my own, stood on a dock, and took in the sight of the crimson sky and the waves beneath. The water was rough and crashed against the rocks, but she was beautiful.

We hit the road again in the morning. After three days of being in the car, we were excited when we started seeing signs for Wisconsin, letting us know we were close.

We stayed at a small beachside motel, but it was so much nicer than a motel. The "rooms" were actually nine white individual cabins with kitchens and BBQs outside. Each had two beds, a fireplace, a TV on the wall, and plenty of rustic beauty.

It reminded me of "Kellerman's" from *Dirty Dancing*. If I could have moved in and never left, I would have.

The motel was a family business owned by a woman named Shirley and run with the help of her daughter, son-in-law, and their children.

Suze, her daughter, was very friendly and welcomed us when we arrived. "I was so excited to get the call that you'd all be staying with us!" she said genuinely. She invited us to join her down on the beach that night to watch the sunset and have a fire with her husband, Dean, and her brother Randy.

We took her up on her offer, bringing marshmallows, chocolate, graham crackers, hot dogs, and buns. They had seats set up for all of us.

We spent the night bonding over stories of where we all come from and what had brought us together.

Suze asked me if I would like to go Yooperlite hunting along the shoreline after the sun went down.

"What on earth is a Yooperlite?" I asked.

Matt already knew what they were because they had them in Michigan, where he was from.

Yooperlites are rocks containing fluorescent sodalite, which causes them to glow under ultraviolet light. They're usually found in Michigan's Upper Peninsula, especially along Lake Superior shores. The name "Yooperlite" is derived from "Yooper," a nickname for residents of Michigan's Upper Peninsula.

We explored the beach, looking for them with a UV light. I didn't find any, but Suze did. When she shone her light on the glowing pebbles, I was amazed.

The next day, Randy checked on us to see if we needed anything. He was in his early fifties, very kind, and wanted to know all about the crossings. I ended up sitting outside with him and immediately knew we'd be lifelong friends.

That afternoon, we went to meet Captain Joe at his marina. He became the second Joe on my team and the first person from Wisconsin.

Superior was roaring when we got there. Inside the marina office, the walls were decorated with photos and nautical ornaments. The table we sat down at had a glass top supported by wood with rope finishing. We were joined by his wife Sarah too. Joe was warm and welcoming, a big guy with long blond hair and big cheeks.

"There's a lot of sheep on the field out there today."

"Excuse me?"

"Whitecaps," he said. Apparently, whitecaps on the water looked like sheep on a field. It was a fisherman's term.

"How fast can you go out there?" he asked. "I don't think the boat can really go slower than three miles an hour."

"I can do that," I said, probably too quickly. I couldn't, but I said I could. I mean, technically, I could go four kilometres an hour.

My team called me on it. "Three miles is nearly five kilometres, Mike," one of them said gently.

"I will go as fast as we need to go out there." We had to make this work.

At the end of the meeting, we decided the weather looked like it would break and be clear in two days, by July 5.

Joe and Sarah were so hospitable and welcoming. Together, we pulled maps of Lake Superior out onto the table and went through the planned routes. Then, we took a walk out to the boat, which would support the team.

It was a fishing boat, and Matt was as excited about it as I was. It was totally different from the other boats. This one had fishing poles and nets hanging off the sides. I'd never been on one before.

That night, we joined Shirley, Randy, Suze, and Dean down on Lake Superior with the waves roaring wildly, breaking on the shore. We spent the night telling stories and singing around the fire, occasionally walking up and down the beach looking for Yooperlites, but I still didn't find any.

* * *

By July 4, the waves were still crashing violently against the shore. I couldn't even imagine going out there the next day, but that was the plan and Captain Joe, Matt, and Captain Keith (collaborating by phone from his home) all maintained that the fifth was the day.

While exploring the town, we stopped at a yard sale. We met Ann Bowman, a local artist in her seventies, and spent an hour chatting with her and looking at her beautiful paintings of the lake in all different seasons. She also showed us the cliff at the edge of her property. It overlooked the lake. I could picture her painting at her easel at the top of the cliff.

I was looking at a blue windbreaker with a white zipper in a mesh bag when she offered to give it to me at no charge. She was selling it for a friend and admitted, "My friend would be very honoured if you wore this on your crossing."

We exchanged hugs and I promised her I would come back before we left to let her know how it went.

After thrifting, we went down to the lake to watch Matt,

who had brought his surfboard, try his luck on the Superior waves for the first time. We sat on the beach, watching him pick up waves and ride them back in again and again and again, only to wipe out whenever he made it close to shore.

My heart stopped every time he was tossed off his board and into the surf. *How on earth could I possibly go out there on a paddleboard the next day?*

That night, we joined the cabin crew once more at the firepit.

Suze and Randy continued peppering us with questions about the next day, almost as if they were the ones going out on the water. And that's when it hit me.

"Would you like to come and be on the boat as part of the team?"

They immediately jumped up and down with excitement. I was excited because they were my friends, and you want friends around you when times get tough.

In the distance, Independence Day fireworks were going off, and we walked along the beach with the UV lights, looking for Yooperlites for the last time.

I'd all but given up when I spotted something out of the corner of my eye. There, surrounded by grey pebbles, was the shimmer of gold and yellow.

I'd found a Yooperlite!

I said goodnight to everyone, went to my cabin, climbed into bed, and sent out a tweet to the Lake Superior Twitter account with a photo. The tweet read: "Please play nice tomorrow when my team tries to cross you."

* * *

When the alarm went off at 5 a.m., I checked social media, and the Lake Superior Twitter account reposted my tweet. There were thousands of likes and comments on the post wishing me and the team well today.

Everything was laid out and ready to go—my wet suit, boots, water gloves, an Edmund Fitzgerald sweatshirt, the windbreaker gifted to me the day before, and my little golden bell pin from the Museum.

The team put me on my liquid diet right from the beginning. We walked down to the water. A dense fog had settled over everything. It was eerie and mysterious and everything I had always pictured Lake Superior to be.

I was so caught up in the fog in front of me that it took a while to notice what I was *not* hearing. For the first time since we'd arrived in town, the lake was silent.

Superior was known for her moods, and we were about to see just how well she would treat us.

Dropped off at my launch spot, I was instructed to paddle to the end of the river and onto a sandbar, which would be the official launch point.

I hugged Suze, Randy, and my team before they all left to meet Captain Joe.

I was on my own, just like the moment I stepped foot into the mental health facility.

I made it across the river without a hitch in about three minutes. On the other side, I climbed up the sandbar, holding my paddleboard. One second, I was fine, and the next, the ground was giving way beneath me, pulling me down. What I had seen as just sandy ground was actually deep muddy water, and I was sinking—all the way up to my thighs. Dread took hold. I clawed at the sand and tried to kick my legs, but nothing seemed to be working. My legs could barely move. The heavy mud was squeezing them, holding me in place.

Is this what quicksand is?!

How could I have managed to nearly drown myself in the first ten minutes I'd spent alone in I-didn't-know-how-long?

I called out to my team for help. I had become used to them being there for me when I was in trouble. No one answered. They were on the boat, a good mile away—well outside of earshot.

I whipped my head around as far as I could, searching for something or someone who could help.

To the left, amongst some trees, I caught a glimpse of a little blue house. It was pretty far away, but I didn't care. I screamed, hoping to get someone in the house's attention. No one heard me.

Okay, Mike. Get your shit together. It's just some muddy water. You can do this.

With sweat pouring down my face, I threw my body forward and dug my elbows into the sandbar, using them as anchors. Instead of frantically scrambling, I forced myself to slow down, and more methodically shimmy my body forward, inch by inch. And it worked.

After minutes that felt like years, I got my legs free enough to crawl awkwardly up onto a firmer patch of ground. I crawled another five feet, just to be sure, patted the sand beneath me to make sure it wasn't going to swallow me again, and threw up.

I don't know if it was the terror of my first (and hopefully only) brush with quicksand, or if it was all the weeks' worth of anxiety that had come before this, but my body evidently wanted the stress and anxiety *out*.

When my stomach settled, I flopped back onto the sandbar with my walkie-talkie and waited. I rested my legs and body while I had the opportunity.

"Mike," a voice came over the radio at the same time I heard the sound of our drone flying overhead. "We're ready, it's go time."

I got on my board and paddled through the fog to the support boat, leaving the cliffs and trees (and quicksand) behind me.

LAKE SUPERIOR | SOLUTION-SEEKING

* * *

That day, Lake Superior was different from Lake Erie and Lake Huron. The fog was dense but the water was like glass. As my paddle cut through the water, I realized something and smiled.

She's behaving.

The winds and the currents that we did encounter, only pushed us closer to our destination. I was travelling at a speed of 7.25 kilometres an hour, which was the fastest I had ever paddled.

We couldn't see around us, but Captain Joe used his GPS navigation system and radio communication to avoid hitting any obstacles.

I knew there were ships out there. Every twenty to thirty minutes we heard the horn of one nearby alerting us that they were there in the fog.

We followed our usual routine. A whistle or bell was sounded every thirty minutes. I'd eat, have a wellness check, be asked how often I was going to the bathroom, how I was feeling, and if I needed anything … I embraced the familiarity of it all.

At 11:30 a.m., the fog cleared. The water shifted to a dark blue. I needed to get rid of clothing as the temperature rose, handing off items to Suze and Randy.

Having Suze and Randy on the boat was incredible. They were as welcoming every time I came over as when we first pulled up to their motel.

At 12:30, the whistle blew. When I came over for food and re-hydration, I was told, "We need to have a talk."

Uh oh. That's never good.

"We have good news, and we have bad news," they said.

The good news was *really* good. We were on track to arrive just before 3 p.m.—seven hours early! The winds and currents had been pushing and helping me. It was incredible. I looked down at my bell pin and smiled.

Then came the bad news.

"We are good for another hour, and then it's going to get rough. We need you to go as fast as we can for the next hour."

"How bad does it look on the radar?" I asked.

Matt simply said, "You need to really push."

I could tell from Matt's reply that the lake was going to get really violent.

I gathered up the strength gained from the previous hours of smooth sailing and, for a straight hour, I paddled as fast as I could. The team cheered me on with whoops and hollers. I went faster than ever before, and soon, I could even see the shoreline in the distance.

That's when the clouds rolled in. The sun disappeared, fog surrounded us, and it got cold fast. I called for a sweatshirt and winter hat as the temperature plummeted.

The water turned on me. Swells picked up, crashing on both sides of my board and my support boat.

I looked over at Captain Joe, and we locked eyes. Worry and dread. That's what I saw.

"Sheep on the field, Captain Joe."

Joe nodded. "Keep going."

I did. I paddled as hard as I could, but I knew everyone could see my energy fading.

I drew upon the resilience and strength that I'd built in past moments of darkness, health trauma, and of course, difficult Great Lake crossings. I drew upon those times when I'd been pushed to the edge, desperate to just give in, but instead, found a way past the impossible and through to the other side. Those times, those memories, gave me a gift that is priceless—the gift of learning what I was capable of.

I fought the waves and focused on Minnesota, the finish line. It's all there was.

"We're close, Mike," someone said from the boat. I'd never heard more beautiful words in my life.

The team was going to go ahead of me once we came around the lighthouse on the pier that was supposedly ahead of us.

I was exhausted from the last hour of fighting. I could feel it in my arms, shoulders, back and legs.

The waves were so big I could only endure them sitting down at this point.

I tried to see the lighthouse they were talking about. All I could see was spray from the turbulent water.

"It's there! Keep going," the team shouted.

I was barely doing one kilometre an hour by then, thanks to the wind blowing us all backwards.

I tried to ignore my screaming muscles when a new pain burned across my chest and down my arms. I knew as well as anyone else what the symptoms of a heart attack were and was immediately scared.

(I was not having a heart attack. My body and mind were reacting to the stress of what it was going through.)

I decided to keep going. I couldn't handle the thought of being pushed backward while having a wellness check, and then having to make up for that lost distance with harder, longer paddling.

A few final pushes later and it appeared. I could see the lighthouse. It was white with a red roof. I could see it and we were getting closer to it. All I could think was *thank God!* Or maybe I should've been thanking the lost crew of the Edmund Fitzgerald.

I let the lighthouse draw me toward it with the promise of safe harbour. I started to make out the silhouettes of people underneath it as I got closer.

When it was time, my support boat veered off and moved ahead. I was now on the safe side of the pier and protected from the angry waters crashing against its other side.

I stood up on my board for the first time in hours and made my way to the shore of Two Harbors, Minnesota.

Now I could see my team waving the Canadian flag

back and forth. It had been attached to the boat throughout the crossing.

"You did it!" I heard them scream. "Number three, baby!"

I shakily got off my board and stepped into a sea of hugs and high-fives before sitting back on the sand to catch my breath.

I could've sworn I heard Lake Superior excusing her last hour of bad behaviour: *I gave you all day, Mike.*

Suze was crying with relief. When I was ready, she helped me get back up to meet the media and people on the shoreline.

Reporters from the local NBC, CBS, and FOX news outlets had their tripods set up facing the water and interviewed me all at the same time, asking questions about what our day had been like.

"She let me across . . . a bit of a fight in the end, but she let me across," I said, nodding toward Lake Superior. "And my team helped me through the hard parts."

I thanked everyone for coming and made my way back to the boat and then back to Wisconsin.

After a violent return trip, a welcomed back hug from Sarah at the dock, and a barbecue I could barely keep my eyes open for, I said good night to everyone and went to bed.

Before crashing, I went online and let the Lake Superior Twitter account know we made it across. I posted a photo the team took of me while out there with the Canadian flag blowing off the side of the boat with me paddling alongside it.

"We made it across Lake Superior today. We did it."

* * *

I woke up to social media blowing up on my phone. The Lake Superior Twitter account re-shared my tweet and sent a congratulations message. There were thousands of likes and hundreds of re-tweets.

I received messages from Jann Arden, TSN broadcaster Michael Landsberg, and from Rick Hansen. Arlene Dickinson of the TV show *Dragon's Den* tweeted out, calling on the Canadian media to cover the story. The mayor of Toronto, John Tory, sent out messages on social media. So did several federal members of parliament and mayors from across Canada.

My phone was filled with messages from my parents, my family, friends, and supporters cheering us on. It was surreal.

Later, we visited Ann Bowman to thank her for her gift and to get a picture so that I could remember her.

We had dinner with Captain Joe, his wife, their daughter, and Shirley, Suze, Randy, and Dean, followed by our last campfire on the beach.

The conversations were filled with stories of the crossing, as seen through the individual lenses of each team member.

By the end of the night I had decided: Superior was my favourite lake.

She would always be part of me.

LESSONS IN SOLUTION-SEEKING

When nothing is going according to plan, the ability to seek out solutions will make or break your outcome. That's true whether you're in the middle of a cold, dark lake, barely able to paddle one more metre forward, or you're building skills for personal or professional goals.

Solution-seeking is a skill that gets better with age and experience. The more you face adversity, and the more times you find a solution and a path through, the more resilient you become.

Through my neurological illness, mental health crisis, and the Great Lakes campaign, I have been faced with finding an answer at times when I essentially felt as if I were drowning.

Here's what I teach organizations who are trying to solve huge problems that, at first, seem impossible:
1. Clearly identify the problem. In our case, we needed to get from point A to point B, and we had no transportation to do so. Plus, the weather was looking terrible for the entirety of our weather window.

2. Brainstorm solutions with the team, welcoming all ideas, no matter how strange they might have seemed. Brainstorming must be a zero-judgment activity.
3. Walk away—or, as in my case, go out for breakfast!
4. Select and implement the solution that will be the most effective. In our case, that was switching lakes and captains.

CHAPTER 10

LAKE MICHIGAN | 4:1
MENTAL HEALTH

The weather cooperated better than we could have ever imagined for our Lake Superior crossing.

Now that we'd conquered the lake I'd feared most, I felt much more confident about the upcoming challenge of Lake Michigan.

As soon as we got back, I started seeing messages from people in Ontario. Signs had gone up in front of schools, libraries, and city halls. "Let's Go, Mike!" they read, directing people to our campaign, showing their support.

I couldn't believe how far we had come. The year before, we hadn't even made it halfway across one. Now, we had three lakes under our belts, and I had a solid team supporting me. I wasn't the same person I'd been a year ago. I felt as if I could face whatever was next.

After Superior, we all went home for a short break. We had

been pushing hard, and everyone needed a couple of days to rest and recover.

I was exhausted. But as always, my mind worried about the next plan we needed to make, the next task to complete.

Within two days, I was back to working with the team, looking ahead to Lake Michigan and preparing for what lay ahead in Chicago.

We found a boat for Lake Michigan. Captain Chris, a Chicago-based boat owner who usually rented his boat for parties and events, agreed to captain for us. But there was a catch. Given the long hours out on the water, we needed another captain for safety, just like we had on Lake Huron. This crossing would take just as long, about thirty hours, and no one could handle that kind of time alone at the helm.

We called Captain Jim to see if he'd be willing to come to Chicago with us and assist Captain Chris.

There was a long pause on the other end of the line, and then I heard a loud "Yes!" Jim was in, and his wife, Jane, gave her blessing. Jim would drive down to Chicago the day before the crossing and then head back to Goderich after it was completed.

The drive to Chicago was exciting. I'd been there once before with my family, and of all the American cities I'd visited, Chicago was one of my favourites. The canals, the green spaces, the food, and the sports—it all made Chicago feel special to me.

Matt and Joe drove in from Michigan together. We met in downtown Chicago, near North Avenue Beach and drove together to Michigan, where we would meet up with Captain Chris and Jim. From there, we would begin the Lake Michigan crossing, hopefully ending in Chicago.

> LAKE MICHIGAN is the only one of the Great Lakes located entirely within the United States, bordered by the states of Michigan, Indiana, Illinois, and Wisconsin. It covers an area of 58,000 square kilometres, making it the second largest of the Great Lakes. It is 494 kilometres long, 190 kilometres wide and an average of eighty-five metres deep, with the deepest point being approximately 282 metres.[28]

When we met Captain Chris, he was standing on the top deck of his boat. For the first time during this entire campaign, we had a boat with two decks. He was a quieter guy than Captain Keith and Captain Joe, but he was friendly and professional. He gave us a tour of the boat, showing us the bunks, the kitchen, and where we could prepare food. It was exactly what we needed.

After leaving the marina, we headed to our motel in New Buffalo, Michigan. Driving through Chicago reminded me of an Americanized version of Toronto. It had that bustling city energy, much like home.

This crossing felt different from the others. The turnaround

---

28 Wikipedia Contributors. 2024. "Lake Michigan." Wikipedia. Wikimedia Foundation. September 19, 2024. https://en.wikipedia.org/wiki/Lake_Michigan.

time was short. We knew our weather window, and we had expertly timed everything to move quickly. We were getting good at this.

The next day, we stocked up on supplies, prepping to fill the boat with food and water for the captains and our support team.

New Buffalo was a small beach town, the kind where every other store was an ice cream parlour or beach shop. We secured a slip for the boat at the local marina and arranged for the gas pumps to open early so we could fill up before heading out. Then, we took a walk down to the beach. The place was packed with families playing in the sand, all waiting for the sunset. I wandered over to the lighthouse, the launch point for the next morning.

As I stood there, looking out at the water, I felt the familiar mix of excitement and nerves. The crossing of Lake Michigan was about to begin. The boat was ready. The team was ready. And I was ready—at least, I hoped I was. Tomorrow, we'd find out.

We went for ice cream. The boys were adventurous with their choices, picking fun and quirky flavours, but I stuck to what I knew best—a simple hard scoop of vanilla. I was always a bit of a "plain Jane" when it came to food. The streetlights flickered on, and we knew it was time to head back.

As we made our way back to the van, I lost my footing, fell forward, and landed hard on my right ankle. The pain shot through me instantly.

No! This can't be happening!

My ankle screamed and I thought of the next day's crossing. This was the same ankle that had been injured and waterlogged during the Lake Huron crossing, and now, just as I was beginning to feel stronger, I'd done something to it again.

The guys helped me up and sat me on a nearby bench. I gingerly lifted my leg and rested my foot on my knee, trying to assess the damage. The pain was sharp, and I fought back tears of disappointment and worry. Matt ran back to the ice cream shop and grabbed some ice, using it as a cold compress to keep the swelling down. For ten minutes, I sat there, my ankle elevated, my mind racing with worry.

Eventually, I limped back to the van with the guys supporting me, and we headed back to the motel. Everyone was concerned, asking me if I needed anything, but I didn't say much out of fear. Inside, I was panicking.

How can I possibly paddle tomorrow?

Will I be forced to do the entire crossing on my knees, or worse, sitting down on the board?

I barely slept that night, tossing and turning as the pain kept me awake. Each time I shifted in bed, the ankle would remind me of the fall.

By the time the alarm went off in the early hours of the morning, I was exhausted. But the pain, while still present, had lessened. I cautiously put pressure on the ankle, testing it out, and to my surprise, I could walk without too much difficulty.

The team knocked on my door, handing me my first feeding of the day, a water bottle filled with carbohydrate powder, water, and a splash of Kool-Aid. This was the routine now—fuelling up for the long, gruelling hours ahead.

The van was packed by 4:30 a.m., with the guys doing most of the heavy lifting so I could save every ounce of energy for the crossing. We arrived at the marina by 5 a.m. to see the boat pulling in, driven by Captain Chris, with Jim helping him tie the ropes to the dock.

It was good to see them again, and we greeted each other with hugs and quick hellos as we loaded the containers of supplies onto the boat. Matt then drove me over to the lighthouse, where I would launch.

While the captains filled the boat with gas, a reporter named Mike from WGN Chicago arrived. He had driven an hour and a half from the city to meet us in New Buffalo, and I was surprised—and grateful—that he had made the trip so early in the morning.

Mike interviewed me, asking about the previous crossings, the weather conditions we expected for the day, and what I was most looking forward to once we arrived in Chicago.

I smiled and told him, "Honestly, a hot shower." After three lakes and countless hours on the water, I had learned to appreciate the small comforts that came after the hard work was done.

As we wrapped up the interview, I said goodbye to Mike

and thanked him again for coming out. Then, it was time. I picked up my board by the side handle and walked into the water once more, feeling the familiar rush of nerves and excitement. This was our fourth Great Lake, and though I was exhausted, I knew we were nearing the end.

Just two more to go. I can do two more.

The wind was on our side that morning, hitting us from the front but not too hard. We kept a steady pace, and within two hours of launching, I could already see our target in the distance. The Willis Tower, formerly known as the Sears Tower, stood tall, some seventy kilometres away, its 110 stories cutting into the horizon. It was reassuring to see Chicago in the distance, and I knew that as the day went on, more of the skyline would come into view.

It was hot, the temperatures climbing into the high twenties, but the boat's music and the banter from the crew kept me going. To prevent myself from getting bored, I changed positions in relation to the boat, either beside it or in front of it. I avoided going behind—it had started feeling too much like I was chasing something I could never quite catch.

By 3 p.m., the wind began to pick up. The team told me I needed to push harder now, to cover as much distance as possible before the wind made it too difficult. The outline of the Chicago skyline was becoming clearer, but the wind was growing stronger by the minute. I was frustrated, not just with the weather, but with myself. I was tired, worn out from weeks of paddling, and it felt like everything was a struggle.

By 9:30 p.m., the team gave me a headlamp, strapping it around my head. The sky was painted with beautiful sunset colours, perhaps the most stunning we had seen on any crossing. The team came out to the front of the boat to take photos, appreciating the moment. And then we moved forward, paddling into the horizon.

At 2 a.m., I could barely keep my eyes open, and every paddle stroke felt like someone had pranked me by attaching a sack of wet sand to the blade. The city lights flickered in the distance, teasing me, but we weren't there yet. The team, sensing my struggle, came out onto the boat's deck, playing music and sitting where I could see them. They wanted me to know I wasn't alone in this, even though it felt like I was.

By 4 a.m., Captain Jim shouted from the boat, telling me to look behind us. I turned and saw a massive ship, about eight hundred metres long—a "laker," as they call it—crossing behind us. "That ship moved for you," Jim said with a smile. "They called on the radio and said they'd move so you wouldn't have to." That small act of kindness from the crew of that enormous ship energized me, reminding me that people were rooting for us, even out here on the water.

That energy was immediately put to the test when the wind picked up again, forcing me to paddle sitting down for the next

LAKE MICHIGAN | 4:1 MENTAL HEALTH

few hours. Under the darkest of skies, my mind began playing tricks on me, leading me to believe I was utterly alone. My mind started spiralling. I couldn't shake the thought, "This will never end. We'll never make it."

They were catastrophic thoughts that mirrored the mental health struggles I'd faced in the past, the feeling of being trapped in something that had no end in sight.

Joe, our crisis management guy, was sent out to sit at the back of the boat with a light beam on me, guiding me through the night, just as he had during the Huron crossing. We played games and talked about life, trying to distract me from the pain and exhaustion. "You've got this," Joe would say, again and again, trying to keep me focused on the finish line.

Despite Joe's help, I was still sinking. So at 4:30 a.m., the team played a message for me from my coach, Jonathan, in which he said, "If you are listening to this, you are at the hardest part of the crossing . . . Remember, you are doing something special, something no one has ever done before." Hearing his voice somehow made my body feel lighter. Even my paddle felt lighter.

As the sun began to rise, I saw the skyline clearly now. The buildings of Chicago were right there in front of us. I was awake, alert, and ready to finish. The hardest part was over, and we were so close.

By 8 a.m., as we made our final approach, three paddleboarders came out to meet me, cheering and calling out my name as they paddled alongside me. I waved back, grinning from ear to ear.

A Chicago Marine Police boat joined us, escorting us the rest of the way to North Avenue Beach.

When I finally stepped off my board and onto the shore, my team was there to catch me. We had crossed our fourth Great Lake. I looked back at the water, seeing the paddleboarders still out there, smiling and clapping. I walked over, fist-bumping them before sitting down on the sand to catch my breath.

Jim grabbed my board, and it disappeared as I was whisked away to meet with reporters from NBC, ABC, FOX, and the *Chicago Tribune*. They asked about the crossings, the team, and what had gotten us through the last thirty hours. I was happy to answer, but my physical strength was shattered, and you could see it in my face and posture.

Once the interviews were done, I headed to the public bathroom to finally take off my wet suit. After thirty hours, it was a mess, and I had no intention of ever wearing it again. I stuffed it into a plastic bag, tying it up like toxic waste, and vowed to deal with it later.

Back at the hotel, I was put straight to bed. The plan was to let me sleep through the day, and we'd celebrate later that night. I took a long, hot shower. I was too tired to stand for it, so I sat in the tub and let the hot water wash away the sweat and exhaustion.

Crawling into bed that afternoon was the best feeling in the world. I was asleep within seconds.

* * *

When I woke sometime later, I saw a chicken burger and fries sitting next to me. It was cold but still good enough to take a few bites before falling back asleep.

* * *

That night, the team and I headed out for a well-deserved celebration. Captain Chris had recommended a pizza place in the south part of the city. Over deep-dish pizza, we recounted the crossing and shared stories. They told me about how they almost gagged when they opened the cooler where I'd stashed the wet suit earlier. We all had a good laugh, calling it the "toxic cooler" and deciding I should just burn the wet suit.

After dinner, we walked through downtown Chicago, taking in the sights. We ended up at the top of the John Hancock Building, having drinks and enjoying the 360-degree views of the city. It was a perfect way to end the day.

The following morning, we walked to a store to grab a newspaper. I wanted a copy of the *Chicago Tribune* for my dad. As we entered the store, someone I didn't know looked at me and said, "Congratulations!"

I thanked him, a little surprised, and then picked up the paper. There, on the front cover, was our story: "Disabled Athlete Crosses Lake Michigan on Paddleboard."

We had made the front page of the *Chicago Tribune*.

THE BEACONS WHO SAVED ME

My team saved me from Lake Michigan, even though she was doing her best to beat me. It had taken over thirty people (logistics coordinators, support crews, navigation and weather experts, copywriters, graphic designers, land crews, and more) to make the Great Lakes campaign happen, but the ones on the boat in 2022 who were supporting me in the darkness, waves, currents, wind, cold, and illness—those people saved me and this call-to-action campaign for change more times than I can count.

To be a beacon of light for someone who is lost—to truly provide safe harbour—takes providing emotional and psychological support.

To sit with another human being in their hardest times, championing them to keep moving forward when they've got nothing left to give, that is the work of a Lightkeeper. A beacon.

They took the light off of me and lit a path out of the dark for me. It is something all of us can do. If every year, one in five Canadians gets lost in the mental health crisis, the other four of us could take a lesson from my Lightkeepers in those Great Lakes. Let's take the spotlight off the ones with the "problem," and light up a path to support.

There is power for exponential change there.

CHAPTER 11

LAKE ONTARIO | TOGETHERNESS

The time between the fourth and fifth crossings was the longest stretch of recovery for both my team and me. Not only were we tired, but many of the team members had been sacrificing time with their families and kids to be part of this journey, which took an additional emotional toll. I could see it in their faces and hear it in their voices—we were running on empty.

Burnout is a term thrown around a lot, but the real weight of it is felt physically, emotionally, and mentally, all at once, in a twisted tangle caused by prolonged stress and overwork. This wasn't just the weight of five marathons. This was the heaviness of two relentless years of training, preparing, and being in constant fight-or-flight mode, going from one challenge to the next, trying to reach that final finish line.

Now, the end was in sight.

This last leg was the rematch I'd been waiting for since I was pulled out of the water nearly a year before—*Lake Ontario*.

It was scheduled for the second weekend of August.

This time would be different. We had a plan. We had a route. And, for the first time since I started this journey, the finish line felt like it was within reach.

My team was notified that arrangements had been made, and the Prime Minister of Canada, Justin Trudeau, would be on shore when I arrived. That news alone gave me a boost of adrenaline. The fact that the highest official in the country would be there to mark the end of this journey was incredible. It wasn't just for me—it was recognition for the entire team, for the organization, and for the cause we were supporting.

The boat for this crossing had been secured months in advance, the team was assembled, the dates were locked, and the logistics were far simpler than they had been for the previous crossings.

But we still faced one unique challenge—where to land.

Because I used to teach paddleboarding in front of Toronto's harbour with the city skyline as my backdrop, I had requested that we land at Toronto's HTO Park, right in front of the CN Tower. It was a spot that held special significance for me. However, landing there meant we would have to enter Toronto Harbour, a busy and complex waterway. No athlete attempting to cross Lake Ontario had ever landed there for safety reasons.

The logistical maze to make this happen was unlike anything we'd faced. For seven weeks, the team communicated back and forth with the City of Toronto Parks and Recreation Department, Ports Toronto, and the Toronto Port Authority. There were so many forms and permits to be filled out that I half-joked that I'd completed a second master's degree in bureaucracy. It was surreal to think that, despite having taught paddleboarding in that very harbour and regularly bringing clients there, entering the harbour as part of this crossing required navigating a labyrinth of approvals.

When we did get the green light and HTO Park was secured, I knew it was meant to be. Not only would it be visually stunning, but it was deeply personal.

This was where it had all started, and this was where it would end.

* * *

With the logistics squared away, the focus was on the team. Captain Keith and Captain Jim had bonded over the last few months, and Jim, despite already having supported us on two other crossings, offered to join again. I couldn't believe how dedicated he was. Keith, Jim, and Matt were in constant communication, tracking weather patterns, looking at forecasts, and strategizing.

Meanwhile, my days were mostly spent alone at home, trying to recover. My feet were battered from the previous four crossings, and I stayed mostly quiet, conserving what little energy I had left. I knew people probably assumed I was out training every day, but in truth, I was doing the exact opposite.

I needed to be in the best shape possible to give everything one last push, and the only way to do that was to rest and recover.

The media coverage grew on both sides of the border. *People* magazine reached out about doing an interview after the final crossing. I found myself on Fox News, News Nation, and several other outlets in the US and Canada. I'd smile for the cameras, say all the right things for the organization, be overwhelmed by the attention and grateful to raise awareness for a cause that mattered to me, but as soon as the cameras turned off, my face would fall and I'd go back home, straight to the couch to rest. I was running on fumes.

By Wednesday, just three days before the scheduled crossing, it became clear to everyone that the weather wasn't going to cooperate. The high winds and waves predicted for Saturday were a sailor's dream—perfect for windsurfers and sailboats—but a nightmare for paddleboarding, kayaking, or swimming. We had to call it. The team unanimously agreed to delay by one week, pushing the launch date to the following Friday, with the landing on Saturday afternoon.

The change didn't affect the logistics too much. The boat was still secured, hotel reservations were adjusted, and even the agreements for the landing spot held firm. But it did mean the prime minister couldn't be there. That stung. I had been looking forward to his presence, not just for me but for the organization. It was a significant opportunity to shine a light on the youth mental health crisis and the work we were doing.

But then, our logistics team reached out to David Onley, a Canadian journalist and broadcaster who served as the twenty-eighth lieutenant governor of Ontario. He had a profound impact on accessibility and disability rights, advocating tirelessly for a more inclusive society. David made a call that left me stunned. Hazel McCallion, known as "Hurricane Hazel," the legendary mayor of Mississauga, would be there instead. At 101 years old, she was a living symbol of resilience and strength. Within two days, arrangements were made, and Hazel confirmed she would be on shore to welcome us in.

As the new date drew closer, I received messages of support from all over Canada. Every word of encouragement pushed me a little further, quieting the voice in my head that whispered, "You didn't make it last time."

On Friday afternoon, August 19, 2022, I pulled into Whitby Marina at 2 p.m. under a sky of unbroken blue. The sun beat down as Matt, Joe, and Jim arrived, joined by Andrew and Dave, two old friends from high school who had volunteered to help out on the tender (our motorized inflatable Zodiac dinghy used for getting to shore or transferring supplies from ship to shore) during the crossing. We loaded up bins of equipment, food, and luggage, and I took a long, hard look at Lake Ontario.

She was as beautiful and as majestic as I remembered. And

I knew she could turn at any moment. If I had to be out here for seventy-two hours, I would be. Whatever it took, I was going to finish this.

As the boat made its way across Lake Ontario to the American side, the team settled in on the top deck. I looked around, feeling something I hadn't been able to put a label on for some time. It was gratitude. I wasn't just on my own out here. I had support. I had a team. We had created something special. *Together.*

When we got to the American shoreline, it was time to go. Andrew and Dave helped lower the board into the water, and Matt and Jim adjusted my hydration pack. For the first time, I wasn't wearing a wet suit—just black shorts and a light blue surf shirt. My skin could breathe, and it felt amazing.

"This time is different," I whispered to myself. And with that, I pushed off, the boat engines humming softly, and we set a steady pace.

I could see Toronto faintly in the distance. It was a hazy outline, but it was there—and we were coming for it.

As the sun set, the evening turned into a fun night spent with friends. The water was like glass, and we shared stories, laughing as the Zodiac, always filled with a couple of the team members, putted along beside me, keeping me company.

By 10 p.m., the water had turned from deep blue to black. I had never seen the stars so bright. Even in darkness, it was still warm. I paddled on as the quietness of the lake surrounded us.

I heard the first boom of thunder around midnight, and my heart skipped a beat. But it was far off, and there was no lightning.

I didn't say a word to the team for fear of them calling the event for safety.

We kept going.

At 3 a.m., we encountered a massive ship crossing in front of us, its towering silhouette cutting through the darkness. I braced myself as the waves from its wake hit us, rocking the board, but I held steady. For a moment, I enjoyed the challenge, welcoming the resistance.

The sun broke over the horizon at 6 a.m., painting the sky in soft shades of pink and gold. The hardest part was behind us. As the daylight returned, so did my energy. But as I pushed on, the sweetness of the Kool-Aid in my hydration pack turned my stomach. Before I could react, I vomited over the side of the board.

Panic gripped me. If I couldn't keep anything down, I wouldn't be able to continue. I decided to skip the next two feedings, giving my stomach a chance to settle. When I finally resumed, I took it slowly, pausing for longer breaks to let my body adjust.

The Toronto Islands appeared in the distance, their outlines unfamiliar from this angle. As we approached the final stretch, two Toronto Marine Police boats joined us, followed by a fire services boat. It felt like a procession as we made our way into the harbour.

I knelt on the board, the weight of the last twenty-one hours pressing down on me. But when I looked out, I saw paddleboarders and dragon boaters in the water, coming toward us, waving, and calling out, "Well done, Mike!"

I stood up.

The cheers from the crowd at HTO Park grew louder as we approached. Bells, whistles, clapping, and shouts of encouragement filled the air. I stepped off the board, climbed up the ladder, and was embraced by my team, my family, and my friends.

It was over. We had crossed the fifth and final lake.

The cameras flashed, and the microphones were thrust toward me. I hugged my mom and dad, feeling a rush of gratitude and love. Hazel McCallion, radiant in mint green, spoke eloquently about youth mental health. And as the Toronto Fire Boat set off its water cannons in celebration, I knew we had done something truly remarkable.

Together, we had achieved what many thought was impossible. We had crossed all five Great Lakes. We were the first to do so in thirty-four years.

CHAPTER 12

LIGHTHOUSES

In the months following the Great Lakes crossings, my life underwent further transformation, beginning with healing. The physical and emotional toll of the campaign was almost indescribable. I was eternally grateful to have two feet on land. In fact, I decided to stay off the paddleboard for nearly six months as I processed everything that had happened.

The lakes had tested me, pushed me, and showed me what I was capable of. They took me to my limits and then, just when I was about to give up, they brought me back home.

My body was screaming for rest and recovery. I had learned the hard way to listen closely to what my body needed, thanks to Ramsay Hunt syndrome and the Great Lakes campaign.

And so I listened.

I embraced anything and everything that brought me comfort; sweatpants, binge-watching Y&R, food delivery, and sleeping. From beneath my hoodie and blankets, I found joy in the many messages of love and congratulations that came in by email, text, voicemail, and DMs, even though I couldn't bring myself to reply to half of them. I wanted to write thoughtful, heartfelt responses, but I wasn't there yet.

Sometimes I didn't leave the couch for an entire day. And that was okay. My only job was to heal.

After about two weeks, I was able to walk from room to room without getting tired. I was able to reply to messages without struggling to find the words. My strength was coming back fast and I was getting the itch to return to the life I had built for myself.

It was time.

News media channels were eager to get more details about the crossings and what really happened out on the water, and I embraced the coverage for my cause. It was a whirlwind of awareness for mental health and recognition for my team and their incredible efforts. Our names and photos were everywhere across Canada.

The Jack.org team was happy to see the mental health crisis in the spotlight. The awareness and discussions that started because of the campaign were priceless. I was flooded with requests to talk about it. *All of it.* More than one hundred years after mental health was considered a sin and patients were locked up like criminals, here we were having open conversations about depression, anxiety, and other mental health challenges on every conceivable platform.

The right questions were being asked: "What now?" and

"How can we make this better?" and "How can we support those who need it?"

Provincial and federal legislatures acknowledged our campaign. The Mood Disorders Society of Canada honoured me with the 2022 Marg Starzynski Mental Health Leadership Award.

I was asked to share my journey with companies, academic institutions, and government agencies because it turned out that my story and the lessons I'd learned from it were entirely transferable—to other parts of my life, to other people, and to organizations trying to enact change in the world or within their own ecosystems. Mental health was something that mattered to every single person I spoke to.

In February 2024, an email arrived from Andrew Perez, a political commentator and strategist who had followed the campaign from the beginning. He wrote that my journey across the Great Lakes inspired him and had become a beacon for him throughout his own struggles. It meant a lot to me to read his words.

The next major email I received was an invitation that brought everything I had done back to centre—it had all come full circle. The email was from the Canadian Association for Suicide Prevention (CASP) and they were inviting me to be the keynote speaker for the 2024 Annual CASP Conference.

CASP is a national charity that envisions seeing a Canada without suicide. It was launched in 1985 by a group who saw the need to provide information and resources to communities to reduce the suicide rate and minimize the harmful consequences of suicide-related thoughts and behaviours.[29]

CASP was an organization that wanted what I wanted—to help make sure that no one else had to experience the darkness, isolation, or loneliness of depression.

> TO: Mike Shoreman
>
> SUBJECT LINE: Keynote Speaker Invitation: Canadian Association for Suicide Prevention: 2024 National Conference
>
> I'm writing to you today with an invitation to be a keynote speaker at the Canadian Association for Suicide Prevention Annual National Conference being held in beautiful Vancouver, British Columbia, May 29–31, 2024.
>
> The CASP Conference is Canada's premier suicide prevention event that showcases the most current knowledge, trends and practices from the field, and

---

[29] "About Us - Canadian Association for Suicide Prevention." 2024. Canadian Association for Suicide Prevention. August 21, 2024. https://suicideprevention.ca/about-us/.

> attracts researchers, front-line clinicians, people with lived experience, and sector professionals from across Canada.
>
> The theme for this year's conference, "Inspiring Hope Together," emphasizes the power of unity in creating positive change.
>
> As a prominent and tireless mental health advocate we'd love to have you attend our annual conference and speak to your lived experience and extensive advocacy in the mental health and suicide prevention space. Keynote presentations will include a Q & A segment and total a minimum of 70 minutes to a maximum of 90 minutes.
>
> Thank you for considering this presentation request. We look forward to hearing from you and, hopefully, to working together at this year's Conference to inspire hope and create positive change in our communities.

I will admit, the invitation brought tears to my eyes. CASP was referring to *me* as a "prominent and tireless mental health advocate." There were many times during my depression and in the middle of vast waters that I wondered if anyone cared, if any of it would make a real difference. The self-doubt, like the water, came in waves and had the power to knock me down.

To be a keynote speaker at the CASP 2024 Annual Conference was the opportunity of a lifetime.

I re-read the letter, trying to focus on the words as my mind raced ahead, already plotting out the ideas I would share on that stage in front of the four hundred mental health professionals and leaders from across Canada who would be in attendance.

That audience was filled with people I aspired to be. People who made change in the world.

In early March, I met Sean Krausart, CASP's Executive Director, and his right-hand Pat Doyle. Pat told me about the thirty-four years of conferences they have held across Canada, and how the event was designed to bring mental health community leaders and organizations together.

I pitched the idea I'd been working on, which I knew would either be seen as game-changing or unrealistic. I remember forgetting to breathe as I waited for their feedback. It was hard to tell through Zoom what their body language might be giving away. But CASP was all in. The team was excited about the concept.

With just a few months before the conference, I immediately started prepping my presentation, pulling lessons learned from each phase of my illness, my depression, my comeback, and then, of course, the lake crossings and all they entailed.

I wanted the keynote to be perfect. Planning it became a part-time job.

My other part time job consisted of travelling across Canada, speaking to and working with organizations, companies, and academic institutions. With each event I spoke at, I further brought my idea for managing the mental health crisis to life, sharing it and applying it to the circumstances and audiences I spoke to, gaining knowledge from feedback as I went.

My work was fulfilling but also a challenge. During these days, I was either connecting with event organizers or speaking to their audiences. Evenings were spent in hotels, alone. In the past, I would have felt isolated. This time, I looked at the time alone as a gift and used it to write, rehearse, and prepare for the CASP event.

As if that wasn't enough, I did an eleven-minute TEDx Talk that was to be released on or around the time of the conference. The talk featured my focus on flipping the mental health crisis statistic, an idea I planned to share and expand upon at CASP. Delivering the right message meant everything to me.

Just two weeks before CASP, TEDx released my video and it quickly crossed into the top two percent of all TEDx talks released globally. The story was hitting home. For everyone.

Finally, it was May 27, and I was on a plane from Toronto

to Vancouver. It had been six years since I'd been to the West Coast, but instead of Laguna Beach, I was headed to Vancouver.

I stepped out of the airport and took a breath. I soaked it in, permitting myself to live in that moment and absorb the sunshine and crisp, clean air.

I checked into my downtown hotel, bee-lined for my room and was immediately struck by the view before me. Huge windows in my room were a portal to the breathtaking natural beauty of the Pacific Ocean and the mountains surrounding it.

I stood before the windows, revelling in the feel of the carpet beneath my feet, grateful for the strength in my legs and the fact that I didn't have to fight for balance. I allowed myself to acknowledge how far I had come.

The window cast my reflection back at me, and I smiled my slightly asymmetrical smile without hesitation. That in itself was something that, years before, I wasn't sure I would ever do again. I would've bet my life on the fact that nothing would ever get better. I could only feel thankful for the people and support that prevented me from successfully placing that bet.

In that pristine guest room, nature's beauty and my life's possibilities were all I could see. I felt lucky. *No.* That's the wrong word. *I felt strong.*

I was about to educate and inspire people who had spent their lives being beacons of hope for others. And they wanted me to teach them.

It was an honour, and I had every intention of living up to their expectations.

The next day, I woke up early and went for a walk along the waterfront, appreciating the morning views and the grey overcast weather that Vancouver is known for.

It was May 28. My birthday.

The morning was dedicated to attending the pre-conference event entitled "Healing Day." It was a series of workshops led by mental health practitioners and organization leaders—mostly in breakout rooms.

My friend Kristin Light (aptly named), who also worked in the mental health education space, was presenting a workshop that morning. She looked flawless, with her hair done up, wearing a beautiful pink dress. I could see anxiety in her expression and could definitely relate, but when she took the stage, her nerves disappeared and she delivered an informative, humorous, and emotional presentation. Many people from the audience came up to speak with her afterward. I could tell that her talk resonated with them.

She went back to her room to recharge, and I spent the afternoon with my friend Mike, who had driven up from Canmore, Alberta, to see me.

We took the little ferry over to Granville Island. The mountains surrounded us as we crossed the inlet.

Mike and I visited the pizza bakeries and artsy shops before taking an eight-minute gondola ride up to the top of Grouse

Mountain. On a clear day, it is said that the top of Grouse gives viewers the best views of the city of Vancouver, but it was misty that day, so we rode up and into the grey. The only thing I could see through the windows were tall Douglas fir trees on both sides.

At the top, it was clear I was not dressed for mountaintop weather in late May. There was snow on the ground and the air was cold against my bare legs. But I wasn't about to miss the opportunity to explore, reminding myself again how lucky I was to be physically able to do so.

With a borrowed windbreaker and shorts on, we walked along the path, taking in the sights and even visiting the bear sanctuary (home to three rescued bears that live there throughout the year).

We watched an old-fashioned lumberjack show—two men pretended to be lumberjacks, competing for who could chop wood in the fastest and sometimes most ridiculous way possible. The crowd loved it. I loved it. It was light and fun, and it made me laugh.

That's when I realized something: I was on the other side of this. After six long years and all that I'd been through, I could finally say, without a doubt, that I was okay. I felt safe. Through all the struggles, through all the times when I had no hope and it felt as if the pain would never end, I'd made it through.

I kept this thought to myself as we got back on the gondola and headed back down the mountain. This time, as we descended, the sky cleared, and we were able to see all of Vancouver laid out in front of us.

It reminded me that just as the darkness of night eventually becomes the light of day, so can the fog lift right in front of us.

That evening, I sat at a dinner table overlooking the Vancouver waterfront. Sean Krausert of CASP had arranged it so that I wouldn't be spending my birthday alone. There I was, sitting with mentors and new friends, as they shared funny stories, talked about politics, and celebrated life with me.

I smiled, feeling overwhelmed and grateful for the people there—and for the people who helped lead me there.

* * *

The morning of my CASP Conference talk, I woke up filled with excitement. I'd laid my clothes out the night before, including my pristine, ironed shirt. A hot shower refreshed me and I took a pause to sit on the bed for a while, looking out at the water planes as they landed and took off again, flying to destinations unknown.

It was May 29, 2024, two years to the day since I was in Crystal Beach, preparing to attempt the crossing of Lake Erie. This time, I was preparing to give the most important keynote address of my life. I was ready. This was the day.

I spent the morning going over the script a few times, finalizing the order of events, and reviewing my talking points for that afternoon. I've always found the ritual of review and study to be comforting. It helped ease my nerves before they had a chance to take hold.

I said goodbye to the view that had been mine for the last few days and checked out of my room mid-morning since I'd be flying home directly after my keynote presentation.

After morning sessions, I ventured into one of the mostly empty ballrooms with my lunch. A woman turned to look at me, and when our eyes met, I felt compelled to ask if I could join her. I asked her which organization she was from.

"Oh, I'm not with an organization," she said quietly. "I'm from Montreal. I came on my own."

I looked at her in surprise.

"My husband took his life almost a year ago," she explained and I winced, thinking of the pain she must be going through. "When I saw an ad online for this conference about suicide prevention, it felt like a chance to be surrounded by others who might understand what I'm experiencing."

I gave her a hug. There weren't many words that could alleviate what she was feeling, and yet I felt honoured just to have met this woman. "I'm so sorry," I said honestly. "I admire your courage for coming here on your own."

This woman had made a choice. She took action. That first brave step would lead her to her next.

When it was time, I was taken to the speakers' greenroom. I used the time to get myself into the emotional and psychological state required to deliver my message. I said my affirmations and focused on positive self-talk.

By 3 p.m., the ballroom was filled with mental health leaders from across Canada. There were two massive screens on either side of the stage to share my videos and slides while I spoke.

From the side of the stage, I watched as my introduction video played and I could feel my heart beating through my chest. When it finished, Sean Krausert welcomed me to the stage and I made my entrance, using the accessibility ramp. Sean greeted me with a hearty handshake before leaving me at the podium. I began.

* * *

I shared my fight with a rare neurological disease, the dark path that took me down, and how I had only found my way back after asking for help. I talked about the magic in finding my beacons in the dark.

Lighthouses and long-range lights stand sentinel along Canada's rugged coastline—the longest coastline in the world. These steadfast beacons guide ships safely around treacherous shoals and hidden reefs, bringing sailors home through storm and darkness. They are lifelines.

Lighthouses sound fog alarms that can cut through even the thickest mists, aid pilots navigating above, deliver essential weather updates, sustain crucial radio communications, serve as shelters during fierce storms, and broadcast tsunami alerts along the North Pacific coastline. Above all, they "keep the light," casting a beacon to highlight dangerous coastlines and shallow waters, guiding ships safely to harbour.[30]

The first lighthouse I ever saw was the West Pier Lighthouse in Port Dover, Ontario. I was just a child, standing at the water's edge, gazing up at the towering structure. It seemed almost magical—an unmovable guardian against the restless waves. I didn't understand its purpose then, but something about that lighthouse captivated me—a silent promise of safety amidst the chaos.

Over thirty years later, I have come to appreciate the profound power of the lighthouses. They symbolize hope, support, safety, resilience, and unwavering guidance.

The feeling of being lost in the darkness is all too familiar for the one in five people battling mental health challenges in any given year. It can become a vast, enveloping void where direction is elusive, and every step forward feels uncertain.

As I spoke about real and symbolic lessons, I recalled the nights on the Great Lakes when the wind howled, and the waves rose like mountains, pushing against me with relentless

---

30   Canada,. 2024. "Lighthouses in Canada." Dfo-Mpo.gc.ca. 2024. https://www.dfo-mpo.gc.ca/otw-am/lighthouses-phares/canada-eng.html.

force. The cold spray stung my face, and the darkness seemed infinite. On calmer nights, an eerie silence would settle—a profound isolation broken only by the rhythmic splash of my paddle dipping into the inky water and the distant, reassuring whistle from the support boat, a reminder that I wasn't completely alone.

Those moments mirrored my own mental health journey. There were times when I felt I couldn't go on. Giving up masqueraded itself as an easier path, even though I know now that it never is. But then, through the darkness, a distant light would appear. Sometimes it was the beam of a light from my support crew, other times the beam of a lighthouse piercing the night, steadfast and unwavering.

During the countless hours of battling both the elements and my own self-doubt, I contemplated what it meant to be a source of light for others. I wanted my journey—every struggle, every kilometre—to be a beacon for those who felt adrift in their own lives.

I wanted to show that, yes, the journey is arduous, and yes, the nights can be long, and yes, you will doubt yourself and want to quit, and maybe, you will feel like you're alone, but if you keep moving forward, the shore will emerge from the darkness, and you'll find your way home.

Even now, after the campaign has ended, lighthouses remind me of the people who supported me—the ones who stood firm beside me, offering light and hope when I struggled to find it within myself. People like Captain Keith, who had an unshakable belief in the mission from the very beginning, or Captain Jim, who stepped in when we needed help the most, his dedication surpassing all expectations. My team members, my family, and even strangers who sent messages of encouragement—they were all my Lightkeepers, tending the flame, ensuring it never dimmed, and guiding me back when I drifted off course.

* * *

My TEDx talk opened the first eleven minutes of my keynote speech. I took the audience with me through the crossing of Lake Michigan, my journey from darkness to light. I shared the concept of how easy it could be to take the one-in-five mental health crisis statistic and flip it on its head if we empowered the other four in that statistic to become beacons of light for the one who is struggling—showing up for them like lighthouses and the Lightkeepers within them.

I saw smiles and nods in the audience.

From there, I walked through the six-step framework for implementing change, using video, audience demonstrations, and paired activities to maximize audience engagement and entertainment.

Throughout the presentation, I felt waves of overwhelming gratitude for where I was in that moment and what it had taken to get there . . .

The people in this room were my mentors. The legs I stood on were (mostly) balanced and strong. Photos and videos were being shot from various locations and I didn't feel the urge to hide from them. If the world was spinning even slightly, it was more from excitement than dizziness. And my smile, if not perfect, was real.

I could feel my purpose shift at that podium. It was electric. And I knew it was just the beginning. If my message was making an impact in a space like this for change-makers like these, I could do so much more.

I shared insight, tears, vulnerable truths, and my optimism for change. Occasionally I looked past the spotlight to check whether I was losing anyone's attention along the way. But they were still there, hearts open, every step of the way.

We finally came to a slide that said, "Phone Lights On."

"I want all of you to join me in becoming Lightkeepers. I want to see who believes in the power of possibilities of shining their light for each other and for the most vulnerable."

Within seconds, I saw who the leaders were in the room—the first to turn on their lights. First, ten or so lights appeared in the dark ballroom. Then a dozen. Then several dozen. Eventually, the conference room was filled with hundreds of lights, each symbolizing safe harbour.

Everyone in that room became Lightkeepers at that moment. We were going to help take the pressure off those one-in-five people suffering from mental health challenges by leading the way to support, help, light, and safe harbour.

We were all going to rewrite the ending of stories that were just like mine.

And we were going to do it together.

EPILOGUE

In October 2023, the feature documentary *When Hope Breaks Through* was released. It was directed by Matthew Wagner and chronicled the Great Lakes crossings. Matt had captured countless hours of footage from the support boats, from the waterline, and from the sky. The documentary revealed the best moments and the heartbreaking ones. The documentary has since garnered numerous film festival awards. Each time I attend a screening (the doc is still featured regularly at film festivals nearly every month at the time of *Lightkeepers*' first publication), I'm overwhelmed by the audience's warmth—their smiles, their tears, and their shared stories. It's all a humbling reminder of the impact a single journey can have.

I now know that my purpose is not to solve my own battles myself. I have my support system of Lightkeepers. I also know that I can't solve everyone else's battles. But what I can do is hold space, shine a light, and show that it gets better, that you *can* do this even if you just don't know it yet.

I want everyone to know that darkness may be vast, but it isn't endless. Keep paddling. Keep fighting. And if you feel as if you can't go on, look for the light—it might be held for you by a friend, a family member, a stranger, or someone within the community who cares and knows how to help. And after all of that, perhaps, when you've come through your darkness, you will become a beacon—a Lightkeeper—for others, guiding them to safe harbour.

TEDx Talk:

https://www.youtube.com/watch?v=rjgnbrGq30I

RESOURCES

9-8-8: SUICIDE CRISIS HELPLINE

If you or someone you know is thinking about suicide, call or text 9-8-8. Help is available twenty-four hours a day, seven days a week. This hotline offers support that is:

- bilingual
- trauma-informed
- culturally appropriate
- available to anyone in Canada

KIDS HELP PHONE

Call 1-800-668-6868 (toll-free) or text CONNECT to 686868. Available twenty-four hours a day, seven days a week to Canadians aged five to twenty-nine who want confidential and anonymous care from trained responders.

FOR FIRST NATIONS, INUIT, AND MÉTIS PEOPLES: HOPE FOR WELLNESS HELP LINE

Call 1-855-242-3310 (toll-free) or connect to the online Hope for Wellness chat. It's available twenty-four hours a day, seven days a week to First Nations, Inuit, and Métis Peoples seeking emotional support, crisis intervention, or referrals to community-based services. Support is available in English and French and, by request, in Cree, Ojibway, and Inuktitut.

NATIONAL OVERDOSE RESPONSE SERVICE

1-888-688-NORS

- Overdose prevention hotline for Canadians
- Confidential, non-judgmental support for you, whenever and wherever you use drugs

DRUG REHAB SERVICES

1-877-254-3348

This offers free, confidential professional help and resources for drug and alcohol addiction in Canada, as well as referrals for clients seeking support with substances.

ACKNOWLEDGEMENTS

First of all, thank you to "my four." You know who you are. If you hadn't helped light my way, this story would have been very different.

I am forever grateful to my Great Lakes team. You saved me multiple times in multiple ways. When I talk to organizations about the importance of choosing the right team members, I envision each of you and the ways that you showed up for me and for our shared goal of making a difference.

Thank you to the mental health professionals who helped me on my journey, and to the mental health organizations who dedicate their time and resources to making the world a better place.

I would not have healed as well or as fast if it weren't for my physical therapist, Shane, who helped me learn to function in the world again. Thank you for showing me my strength, and of course, for loving the Toronto Raptors as much as I do.

Thank you to my greatest cheerleader, Andrea. You never

stopped encouraging me to keep pushing forward. You were the voice I needed to hear in some of the darkest moments.

Thank you to my publisher, Jenn Goulden, of Entourage Media. You and Chris proved that as long as there's enough coffee in the world, anything is possible. Thank you for helping me share this story with those who need it most.

Special thanks to all those who were part of this story. You had a significant impact on my life and on helping create change in the world.

And of course, thank you Mom and Dad for sharing your extraordinary love and support. I know it wasn't easy, but you never gave up on me.

ABOUT THE AUTHOR

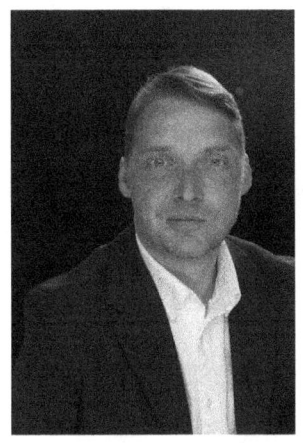

Mike Shoreman is an award-winning mental health leader, educator, consultant and professional keynote speaker. Today, as a record-breaking, disabled adventurer, Mike shatters preconceived notions of what's possible for individuals of all abilities. His articles on mental health and disabilities have been featured in the *Toronto Sun* and in the *National Post*. Mike's Great Lakes crossings crusade for youth mental health has inspired Canadians from coast to coast to coast, helping hundreds of thousands of people.

To learn more about this book, the *When Hope Breaks Through* documentary, or to inquire about Mike's availability as your next keynote speaker, contact team@mikeshoreman.com or visit www.mikeshoreman.com

www.ingramcontent.com/pod-product-compliance
Lightning Source LLC
Chambersburg PA
CBHW051542020426
42333CB00016B/2058